THE TAKE-CONTROL DIET

THE TAKE-CONTROL DIET

A Life Plan for Thinking People

IAN K. SMITH, M.D.

RANDOM HOUSE   NEW YORK

AUTHOR'S NOTE: This book proposes a program of dietary and exercise recommendations for the reader to follow. However, you should consult a qualified medical professional before starting this or any other weight reduction program. As with any diet or exercise program, if at any time you experience any discomfort, stop immediately and consult your physician.

All rights reserved under International and Pan-American Copyright Conventions. Published in the United States by Random House, Inc., New York, and simultaneously in Canada by Random House of Canada Limited, Toronto.

RANDOM HOUSE and colophon are registered trademarks of Random House, Inc.

Owing to limitations of space, acknowledgment of permission to quote from previously published materials will be found following the index.

ISBN 0-375-50730-2
Printed in the United States of America
Book Design by BTD NYC

To Ma, Dana, Noy, and Tristé.

You know what makes me, and you know why I love.

Forever.

PREFACE

There were many reasons why I decided to write this book. As you read through it, many of them become alarmingly clear through my carefully chosen words and anecdotes. However, the first reason that prompted me is personal. In many of the medical columns that I've written for *Time* magazine and the New York *Daily News* and the stories I've reported for WNBC-TV in New York City, NBC's *Today* show, and NBC's Weekend Nightly News, I've spoken fervently about the growing rate of overweight and obesity in our country. Not only is it debilitating our country, but it's truly stealing the lives of Americans and others throughout the world. I have openly and fearlessly criticized gimmick diet books that put helpless and desperate people at risk for serious bodily injury, even death, rather than making use of accepted scientific information.

So when Mary Bahr, an editor at Random House, asked me if I wanted to write something for Random House, I jumped at the chance. For years I've wanted to write health and medical books as well as novels, and out of the blue an editor I had never met was offering me a chance to fulfill a dream and a personal mission. We met promptly, and after our first meeting we had two great book ideas that we thought would do a great service to people. The first, published last year, is called *Dr. Ian Smith's Guide to Medical Websites*, and its purpose is to give Americans a guide that rates ten of the best medical websites for each disease category. Its intention is to help direct people to useful medical information on the Internet and steer them away from those sites that don't have the most current or accurate information.

This book, however, works from a central philosophy of helping you learn about your mind, body, nutrition, and exercise. This knowledge allows you to take control of your life. If you're looking for a book that's offering guarantees about the amount of weight you'll lose in a specified amount of time, then my book is not for you. If you want a magic bullet that will take off those extra pounds, I respectfully suggest you look elsewhere. The only guarantee I make is that this book is the real deal. It respects your sense of integrity and aims to give you a plan not for two months or two years, but one that will change the quality of your life forever.

The take-control diet will challenge you both physically and mentally—something that the journey to success often does. Your part of the contract is being prepared to take and believe in the challenge. If you don't really want to lose the weight and improve the quality of your life, the words on these pages will be hollow and meaningless. However, if you want to make positive changes in your life, you'll have to dig in to what my ever astute brother, Dana, calls those hidden *spaces* that we all have inside of us. These spaces are special reserves of confidence, self-respect, energy, and determination that exist in all of us. If you can tap into them, you'll be well on your way to taking control of life's endless challenges. The golden fuel hidden in these spaces will allow you to turn your life around in the face of failure and criticism and say to yourself, I can do this, because I believe!

It was my aim in writing this book to bring you the latest in scientific research about weight management, a healthy diet, and exercise in an understandable and easy-to-follow manner. I'm concerned about how you manage your weight, because it can have such a tremendous impact on your risk for numerous diseases, self-esteem, and ability to fulfill life's dreams. Please take this work in the following pages not as a bible of information, but as a well-thought-out guide that will empower you to *take control* and live the great life that is your undeniable right.

ACKNOWLEDGMENTS

There are many people who played a major role in helping me bring this book to you: My brother, Dana, who is not only my twin, but my greatest friend in the world, whom I love eternally and who has given me endless ideas about this book and the meaning of life. My mother, Rena, who is as beautiful today as she was that day I first noticed her beauty during a surprise visit she made to my school when I was in fifth grade. You have been and always will be my hero. My cousin, Darius (Fred), who has given me advice and support along the way and who is truly my second brother and great supporter. You were here for me, and I am so grateful. Noy, thanks for making me so happy by bringing so much deserved joy to my mother's life. Tristé, my true love, who has supported, coached, scolded, and enlightened me. How could I have made it without you being there during those long hours? I will always love you. My editor supreme from Random House, Mary Bahr, who has been with me on this project from the very beginning. Mary, you are a writer's dream, and I knew this from the first day we met. My deceased grandmother, who, though not here physically, has been with me spiritually at times when I wondered if this project was too much to bear. I miss you so much. My friends Cards (Jonathan Cardi) and Ron Mitchell—you guys are the true definition of friends, and I shake my head sometimes at how lucky I am that we've had one another for all these years. Leon Carter, much-heralded sports editor of the New York *Daily News*, has been a great sounding board, strong friend, and fearless confidant. Lee, thanks for walking up and introducing yourself at the National Association of

Black Journalists Conference so many years ago. Elisa Zied is the smart and capable nutritionist who helped me put together these menus and count those calories—her expertise and pitching in to help were an important part of this book. Thanks to Jane Freiman, a superb editor of the New York *Daily News,* who gave me my first chance to write a column in a major newspaper. Walter Isaacson, former editor of *Time* magazine, gave me my first column in a major news magazine, the most professional and highest quality of journalism in print media. Jim Kelly, the new editor of *Time,* and Philip Elmer-Dewitt, an assistant managing editor and head of the science section, have supported my endeavors without reservation and made me feel at home at the magazine. Thanks to all of my colleagues who have informed me through all the years and all of my teachers from kindergarten to medical school who have armed me with the knowledge that I share with others. My patients have been instrumental in sharing their stories, taking my advice, and proving that by taking control, you can get your life back. Art Norman, NBC 5 anchorman in Chicago, and his wonderful wife, Ondi, gave me my first start in broadcasting and have supported all of the crazy decisions that I've made over the years—I love you guys! The super-talented Paula Walker Madison (now president and general manager at KNBC-TV in Los Angeles), Diane Doctor, and Dennis Swanson from WNBC-TV in New York City, thanks for allowing me to be a journalist, a job I love with all of my heart, and to continue my important career as a physician. I'm grateful to fellow Harvard man Jeff Zucker who brought me on the *Today* show and introduced me to the grand stage of network television. Last, but certainly not least, thanks to my family not mentioned above who have tolerated me all of these years and made me who I am: Pops (Robert Cherry Sr.), in memoriam the three sisters from little Princess Anne, Maryland—Grandma, Aunt Chris, Aunt Helen—and Aunt Dora Bee, Uncle Bob, Uncle Johnny, Aunt Bettie, Lynn, Aunt Helen Gray, Billy, Uncle Fred, Mr. Brown, Mr. Moseley, Robby, Damian Sr., Oosh (Richard Allen West), little William, Lisa, Walkiris (Keedy), little Damian, Dante—you all are forever in my heart and thoughts!

CONTENTS

PART ONE

HARNESS YOUR THOUGHTS

CHAPTER 1

THE MENTAL EDGE

M ost of my life has been defined by my experiences as an avid sportsman, whether it was playing basketball or swinging the golf clubs. I learned at an early age that what happens on the field of athletic competition is often mirrored in our everyday lives. I was first introduced to the powers that the mind had over the body during my teenage years of playing Pop Warner football. Our most important practice of the week would be Friday afternoon, right before the big game on Sunday. Instead of tackling and hitting one another the way we did during the earlier part of the week, we spent most of the Friday practice perfecting our techniques and analyzing our opponent's expected game plan. Our scouting report often gave us an idea of the offensive plays they'd try to run against us, as well as the defensive formations they'd assemble to stop us from advancing the football.

Friday practices were less about strength and endurance and more about sharpening the mental aspects of our game. The coaches worked us methodically through Sunday's game plan, accentuating most of their points with catchy slogans meant to key our minds into the task ahead of us as well as our physical skills. Coach Murphy had a saying that I heard so often, I would hear it in my sleep before a big game: "Football isn't all about physical prowess. It's 15 percent skill and 85 percent mental." These percentages would change, of course, depending on who was repeating it, but the intended message was equally received—if you wanted to succeed on the football field, your muscles and speed wouldn't do you a bit of good if your mind hadn't mastered the game.

Losing weight requires a major commitment that not everyone is willing or able to make. Depending on how severe the modifications are that you need to make, the physical investment in changing your diet and increasing your level of physical activity can be nothing short of exhausting. Remember, you'll be asking your body to continuously adapt to a lifestyle that will put many of your body's systems in flux. But regardless of how effective a plan you might be attempting to follow, or how physically prepared you are to climb a few extra flights of stairs a day, if your mind isn't in the game, your efforts are doomed before they even get under way.

With the exception of extreme gimmicky diets, much of the science behind weight management programs is the same. Decrease the amount of calories you consume and increase the amount of calories you expend and those billions of fat cells will begin to shrink. Regardless of how fancy the language an author uses or how complicated a formula he or she offers, it's your mind that gives you a major advantage. The beauty of our minds is that they are all different, and the way we process information becomes the individualism of our identity. It would be so much easier if I could prescribe a program that trains your mind to take on the future rigors of a weight loss regimen. The truth, however, is that you must find your own way, one that works for you and makes you feel comfortable. Who knows your mind and body better than you do? I simply offer a few areas of concern and thoughtful advice that you might want to incorporate while developing the winning strategy.

MENTAL TOUGHNESS

*The body fails before the mind, but if the mind is strong enough,
it can resuscitate it.*

DANA O. SMITH

Many things we attempt in life have attached to them a set of prerequisites. If you're applying for a particular job, the company will list the work and educational experience requirements. This same idea of prerequisites transfers to the task of losing weight and making lifestyle changes that will last forever. At the top of the list is a requirement that before beginning any program, your mind is sharp, focused, and up to the arduous task that lies ahead of you.

My brother and I were discussing the prerequisites of anyone heading into battle, whether it be military, athletic competition, or weight loss. We decided that the prerequisite they all shared was the need to have a tough mind, able to charge the body when it felt it couldn't go any farther. Each battle can present its own obstacles, but to reach victory, a participant must be able to mentally overcome any challenge that waits ahead.

Dieting programs, specifically those like mine that advocate fundamental changes for lifelong benefits, are full of obvious and hidden obstacles that crowd the path to victory. Whether it's going over, around, or through these potential stumbling blocks, you're going to need a mental edge to help you navigate the pitfalls. Many people who read diet books brush up on important nutritional facts, such as unsaturated, low-fat foods are healthier than the saturated, high-fat foods. This knowledge, however, means nothing if your body begins to rebel against the changes in your new diet and exercise program. This is where the mind takes over and becomes the savior. If it's properly trained for battle, it's prepared to carry on when exhaustion and frustration have paralyzed you. The mind is that weapon in your arsenal that you can rely on when all other systems fail.

One of my favorite things to do is read the stories of successful people, whether it be in business, Hollywood, or sports. I'm captivated by the strategies they've implemented that have catapulted them above their competition. Most of these stories share certain themes, and mental toughness is one of them. Famous author John Grisham had his original manuscript rejected more than a hundred times by agents and publishers, but it was his mental toughness and conviction in the strength of his work that allowed him to withstand the barrage of criticisms and hold out until it was accepted. Not only was it eventually accepted, but *A Time to Kill* topped the best-seller lists for weeks and was made into a top-grossing movie.

This is the mental toughness that you'll need if your real goal is to attain long-term weight loss and lead a healthier life. Confidence is a natural by-product of this toughness, the belief that regardless of how tough the battles that lie ahead, you'll be able not only to survive, but to surge forward with a determination that nothing and no one will stop you.

REASONS FOR WEIGHT LOSS

Often the reason why you choose to do something can be the most critical factor in your ability to succeed.

There are hundreds of reasons why millions of people reach the decision that it's time to lose weight. The first step, of course, is actually looking in the mirror and honestly admitting to yourself that you need to lose the weight. Your physician or a loved one might tell you repeatedly that it would be important if you lost the weight, but it won't matter at all if you don't truly believe it. Losing weight isn't an easy endeavor; in fact, for many it could be one of life's most difficult tasks. Succeeding will depend largely on the level of your commitment and your ability to persevere when you're tempted to return to your old bad habits.

One of the biggest mistakes dieters make is that they lose weight for others and not themselves. I've talked to several people who've said they're losing weight to make others happy, whether it's a child who's embarrassed by his girth or a loved one who no longer desires a physical interaction because the excess weight is a turnoff. It's great if others are also happy about your decision to lose weight, but you are the primary person who must be pleased. Tying your satisfaction to the approval of others is an unpredictable situation that often ends in failure. The weight must come off because you think it needs to and because you realize its important benefits.

How many times have you said or heard others say, "If I could only lose five to ten pounds by the wedding"? How about this one: "I need to take off another fifteen pounds to get into the clothes I bought last year"? While losing weight and being able to fit into your favorite clothes or feeling good about yourself at a wedding are important, the problem is that you're making an investment in short-term goals. Once the wedding is over or the clothes are no longer in style, many people are no longer worried about what the scale reads and gain the weight back and then some. Once they've lost their motivation—which was event-specific—the drive to lose the weight disappears.

Instead, a better approach to losing weight and keeping it off forever is to look at weight loss as an important change in your overall life. Modifying your diet to make it healthier and increasing your level of physical activity are adjustments that you should incorporate for the rest of your life. People who decide that they want to lose weight because it will make them healthier, allow them to live a better quality of life, and help them live longer are more likely to not only lose the weight, but keep it off longer. These aren't the crash dieters trying to fit into a bikini for summer; rather, these are people who are fed up with being overweight and realize that making these lifestyle adjustments will provide them with lifelong benefits.

I remember speaking with one of my patients who had lost thirty pounds in just a few months. I was interested in what plan she followed to lose the weight, but I was more captivated by her reason for losing it. "After years of trying all of these diet plans and attempting to lose weight to make others around me feel better, I finally decided I was going to lose weight to make myself feel good. I was having pain in my knees and suddenly I was a diabetic, and it all was connected to being overweight." I was even happier that she had lost the weight not on some gimmick diet, but through a commitment to eating fewer calories and making exercise a higher priority in her life. Not only did she eventually lose another twenty pounds, but she also kept it off and became more in tune with her body and her unique relationship to food.

VISUALIZATION

Most people still remember the tremendous talents of former Boston Celtic great Larry Bird. This legendary basketball player amazed competitors and fans alike by his mastery of the game despite the fact that he lacked the physical prowess of other athletes. He couldn't jump, his ball handling was suspect, and he was slower than anyone on the basketball court. What he could do, however, was shoot with a marksman's deft accuracy and refuse to give up even when his team was inevitably facing defeat. During his NBA reign, Bird revealed very little to the media about the secrets of his success, but in a rare moment of openness he said something that I'll never forget. Bird admitted that he played each game several times in his mind—from the opening buzzer to the last shot—before he even stepped onto the court.

The world finally got a glimpse into the mind of one of basketball's greatest players. We soon learned about how his pregame "visualization" translated into his ability to stay one step ahead of almost everyone else on the court. How was he able to always find the open man to pass to? Why did he always seem to know which way the ball was going to bounce? How could he beat others to the basket when he moved as though his feet were stuck in quicksand? It all traced back to his ability to visualize the game and see things that others couldn't.

This visualization can be a tremendous benefit to dieters before they even make the first behavioral modification. It could be a tremendous psychological and practical boost as you imagine yourself changing your dietary choices to healthy fruits and vegetables. Picture yourself stepping on the scale on a weekly basis and finding your weight to be one or two pounds less than it was last week.

You must also, however, visualize the bad times when you can't resist the temptation of a deliciously rich, sugary dessert. Watch yourself eat the entire dessert, then imagine how disappointed the lapse in your willpower will make you. Realism is important here, and you must concede that losing the weight won't be a simple act of wishing the weight away and the scale responding. Instead, imagine two weeks of consistent weight loss, then a week where your weight stays the same. The big focus is on that fourth week and whether you're mentally prepared and physically capable of maintaining a regimen that will continue to burn the calories and pounds.

Arguably the most important reason to be emotionally prepared is to handle those periods of weakness as well as the minor failures that you're likely to encounter. Most people who have attempted dieting will tell you that the easiest part of any weight loss program is the beginning. I've spoken to many patients who've lost so much weight the first couple of months of dieting that they couldn't understand why people made such a fuss about weight loss. Then they hit the infamous "plateau," where the pounds stop coming off and the scale seems to be stuck at the same number.

It's at this critical juncture that mental toughness is an absolute must. You've come to the proverbial fork in the road, and if you're not emotionally grounded and psychologically prepared to stare down temptation until it whimpers away, then you'll take a turn down the road of weight gain. Unfortunately, many people are so frustrated by this juncture, and so overcome with disappointment that the weight is no longer burning away as easily, that they throw their hands in the air and once again eat at will and spend less time participating in physical activities. We'll discuss more on setbacks later in this chapter.

LOSING WEIGHT ISN'T EASY

Bad habits are hard to break, and good ones are hard to form.

If anyone tells you that weight loss is easy, walk away. It's true that some have an easier time than others, but losing weight will certainly not be the easiest thing you attempt in life. In fact, it's going to be downright difficult. You're going to be making demands on yourself to make lifestyle changes, which for some can be quite dramatic. If you've lived a life of eating three thousand calories a day full of chocolate-chip cookies and potato-chip snacks, it's not going to be easy to reduce or eliminate these goodies from your diet. If you spend a majority of your time sitting on the couch watching television or using the computer, then incorporating more exercise and/or physical activity could come as a shock.

If losing weight were such an easy task, there'd be no need for this book or the thousands of others that have come before mine. Weight loss experts would be looking for another specialty and financial analysts wouldn't be calling it a multibillion-dollar industry. The truth, however, is that this industry has been built on the weaknesses, insecurities, and failures of decent human beings who find themselves eternally hopeless in the battle of the bulge.

My mother's numerous attempts and failures to lose weight have been the greatest confirmation for me about how difficult it is to lose weight and keep it off for an extended period of time. My mother is the strongest and most determined person I've ever met. A single mother in the late 1970s and 1980s, she persevered through miraculous hardships so that we could have opportunities to one day succeed in life. I remember as a teenager her constant battles to find a diet that could take off the pounds, satisfy her hunger and tastes, and not cost her a fortune. (The strangest thing about it all was that she, like many other women, really didn't need to be on a diet. She was in great physical shape and great looking as well. I can't count how many times strangers thought she was our sister.)

Even with her ironclad willpower, however, she never found that combination or special program that worked for her. Like millions of others, she also spent a small fortune on these gimmick diet books, miracle supplements, and specially prepared meals that she popped into the microwave. It took years of failures and disappointments before she finally realized that to lose weight successfully , she'd have to stop relying on a magical pill to burn the fat away or some strange eating regimen that eliminated sugar from her diet. Despite all my efforts to teach her the truth about weight loss, it took her failures to help her see the light. She threw away all of those diet books and complicated charts and tables and told me that it was going to take a personal commitment to herself and the same discipline that she had used in other aspects of her life. It took every ounce of willpower in her body to say "no" to foods packed in calories and "yes" to invitations from her colleagues at work to walk a brisk mile during her lunch hour.

People who begin weight loss programs with the idea that it's going to be an easy endeavor have almost prematurely sealed their fate. Their mind-set is already programmed to see the pounds come off with little effort. The first three or four pounds might disappear easily, but when they're unable to go beyond that, they're stuck. They're not mentally prepared to make the necessary lifestyle adjustments that are required to lose more weight. They eventually abandon their weight loss plan, unaware that accepting its difficulty from the beginning would've given them a better chance of continuing on rather than turning around when they hit that first bump in the road.

REALISTIC EXPECTATIONS

Most people who decide to lose weight fail before they even start because their expectations are completely unrealistic and they are soon defeated by disappointment. If you're twenty or thirty pounds overweight, you must realize that it's likely taken you years to accumulate these extra pounds. Yet, you post a New Year's resolution that says you'll shed these pounds in a matter of months. I think most will agree that it's much easier to gain weight than it is to lose it. This, then, begs the question Why would people think that they can lose weight faster than they gain it? The simple answer: Most dieters begin their weight loss programs committed to burning more pounds than they are capable of or more than what is considered a safe amount.

According to the National Institutes of Health and other professional organizations that address weight loss issues, weight loss should be gradual and should not exceed more than one to two pounds per week. While we think of losing weight as just shedding excess fat, it's important to remember that the internal mechanisms of weight loss are complicated and cause a disruption in the body's homeostasis, or environmental stability. Losing weight at faster rates might be more beneficial to achieving your personal goals of reaching a desired size faster, but the resulting cellular alterations can be unsafe and lead to health complications.

It's also important to understand the numbers of weight loss. One pound is equivalent to 3,500 calories. If you require a 2,500-calorie-per-day diet to maintain your current weight, then that means you'd have to reduce your calories by 500 a day to lose 3,500 at the end of seven days. This, of course, doesn't take into account the added boost in calorie expenditure you'd receive by also increasing your level of physical activity, but it does demonstrate how difficult it can be to lose weight through strict calorie reduction. Someone trying to lose two pounds a week would need to reduce the week's caloric intake by 7,000, which means shifting from a 2,500-calorie-per-day diet to 1,500. For many people, a reduction of this size not only is difficult to achieve, but could result in the deprivation of important minerals, vitamins, and other nutrients.

It's important to be extremely careful and clear about the weight loss goals that you set. If you're trying to lose weight for health benefits, studies show that a loss of 10 percent is enough to see changes in certain health indicators such as blood pressure, diabetes risk, and heart disease risk. While it's optimal to attain a weight that's within normal range, the reality is that everyone isn't going to be able to achieve this. However, this 10 percent figure should be the absolute minimum that you strive to achieve.

Still, if you have an ideal weight in mind, don't be afraid to set that as a goal. Realize, however, that most who lose weight and are able to keep it off lose only between 10 and 20 percent of their current body weight. So if you're 200 pounds, you can expect to lose between 20 and 40 pounds. Instead, you might want to lose 70 pounds to drop to a weight of 130. In that case, you must realize right from the beginning that this is going to take a lot of effort and dedication. It's not that you should plan to fail, but you should plan to meet setbacks along the way. Your determination and lifestyle changes will ultimately decide if you're able to reach this lofty goal.

Most diets and their authors sell their plans with an overabundance of optimism, trying to convince you that if you simply follow their program with determination, you'll realize the weight loss that they promise. Optimism is a must for anyone who embarks on a journey to make life-altering adjustments in diet and physical activity, but this must be mixed with a healthy blend of realism. While we all are individuals and have our own track history to help predict the future success of our behavioral modifications, it's important to consider trends that have been noted in the population at large.

Most studies looking at modern weight loss programs show that many people can lose as much as fifteen to twenty pounds in a year's time. This, unfortunately, is the easier part. The number of people who maintain this double-digit weight loss over five years is less than 10 percent. According to some surveys, only five in one hundred people who join commercial weight control programs actually reach their weight goal, but it's unknown how long it's taken them to reach their success or the amount of times they had to re-enroll before they finally hit the mark. The most dismal statistic often quoted about the failure of weight loss programs is that at least half of all dieters not only regain the weight they had lost, but pack on even additional pounds. If the changes one makes to one's diet do not become second nature, weight gain begins as soon as one has achieved one's goal and feels free to go off the diet. Many diets promote dietary restrictions that are simply unsustainable in the long run, so it is natural that someone would return to old eating habits.

When setting your weight goals, there are many variables you should take into account, and understanding the general history of relatively minimal success that accompanies commercial weight loss programs is an important consideration. That's why your goals must move beyond a weight target into the area of life goals. Eating healthier and increasing your physical activities must be imperatives to satisfy not simply an aesthetic goal, but the goals of improving the overall health and functioning of your body so that you can live life to the fullest. A large reason for this is the frequency with which people cycle on and off diets and the overwhelming sense of failure people have when they don't lose that "guaranteed" amount of weight.

One of the major disappointments that people encounter when losing weight is that what they expected to gain from the weight loss doesn't happen to the degree they had hoped. Some people who have been heavy all of their lives and have been chronically ostracized through social exclusion hope that losing weight will bring them social inclusion. It might be true that people will make less fun of a more normal-size person and behave in a more socially gracious manner, but betting that a life of exclusion and embarrassment will be reversed by weight loss is a gamble not worth taking.

People who are mean and small-minded enough to exclude someone for his or her physical appearance are unlikely to change their petty and immature behavior because of that person's alteration in weight and appearance. In fact, when dieters reach that target weight yet don't collect the rewards they hoped it would bring, the spiritual and psychological disappointment only serves as a trigger to undo all that has been done. The disappointed no longer find value in their long sacrifice and hard work and thus return to the bad habits of overeating, consuming unhealthy foods, and finding themselves engaged in more sedentary behaviors.

Your first commitment must be to losing weight for you and only you. This sounds selfish, and it should, because you're the one who must cut back on those favorite between-meals snacks. You'll be the one taking more flights of steps and turning down car rides so that you can walk and kick-start your metabolism. The work will fall squarely on your shoulders, as should the satisfaction. Dieters who tie their own satisfaction to external approval often find themselves in a cycle of hope and disappointment.

FIND SUPPORT

There are those dieters who have lost a tremendous amount of weight and have been able to keep it off without any assistance from friends, loved ones, or professional help. Through a system of self-determination and self-reliance, this small, unique group is able to fight alone and win. But for most people, it's critical to have some type of support system in place to help maintain a rigorous nutritional and exercise program.

Support can come in many forms, but many people who have dieted successfully often talk about how much easier it was to have a friend who also was trying to shed pounds. I recommend finding a dieting buddy, preferably someone who's taking part in a similar program, or at least a program that has at the heart of its philosophy healthier eating and more exercise. It's much easier to commiserate with someone who also must cut down on the number of chocolate-chip cookies or take the time to walk up two flights of stairs instead of taking the elevator.

A diet buddy, however, becomes more than just someone who's there when you just can't resist the urge to raid the fridge. They're also there when you do your weekly weigh-in and find that you've lost yet another pound. Other people might shrug their shoulders indifferently if you were to bound into the office or a meeting of friends and share that you lost a pound. You can bet the farm that the reaction will be a lot different when you reveal this to someone who's also in the trenches, aware of the amount of sacrifice and dedication it took to lose that one pound. Your friendship begins to transcend the normal bond that friends often form—now you've connected on a whole different emotional and spiritual level as you work together toward a common goal.

Support doesn't only mean someone else who's dieting or has tried one. Weight loss experts have found that forging a new friendship or enhancing an old one can be an important distraction. Your energy and activities can now be directed toward something other than worrying about your next meal. In fact, you might be even more inclined to participate in additional physical activities, whether it's walking in the park or joining a gardening club. The busier you are and the more

your schedule is occupied by activities unrelated to food, the less opportunity there is for you to be tempted by unhealthy, fattening foods and sedentary activities such as watching TV.

Some people are more comfortable with structured group interactions that occur among people trying to reach the same outcome. The paradigm that many others have followed over the years because of its amazing success is Alcoholics Anonymous. There are thousands of local and national organizations comprised of people who are weight and health conscious and trying to make changes in their lives that are often too difficult to manage alone. You might find that these programs work for you, if for no other reason than they serve as positive reinforcement for what's good behavior and conducive to attaining your long-term goals.

There is no single best support mechanism for everyone who's trying to make these important lifestyle changes. You know yourself better than anyone else, and you can remember the times when you had to tackle a tough issue, whether it was the recent passing of a friend or loved one or difficulty in a personal relationship. Some find comfort in speaking with their priest or a community leader, while others are fortunate enough to have a loving family and network of friends who can provide the support.

Many people feel that if they seek help or support from others, they are displaying a weakness. In fact, reaching out is more a sign of your strength and willingness to access the necessary systems that will help you achieve your goals. No one gets extra credit for struggling alone, and if your goals are reached, there's no one standing at the front of the line with a medal for those who've done it on their own. Help isn't a bad word, but being afraid to use it can often lead to bad things.

DO YOU HAVE A FOOD ADDICTION?

Many people who are overweight and have been unsuccessful at losing the excess pounds for a long period of time have likely been unaware of their true enemy—food addiction. Just as one can develop a dangerous and uncontrollable addiction to drugs or alcohol, the same can develop for certain foods. Overcoming a food addiction can prove equally challenging and requires the help of someone who has an understanding of these illnesses and can support one's determination to make it better. Getting your food addiction properly diagnosed by a physician or a nutritionist, and, in addition, a psychologist would be the first necessary step before you could expect to successfully begin a weight loss program.

Experts who treat food addicts characterize this addiction as a disorder marked by preoccupation with food, its availability, and the anticipated pleasure from its consumption. Patients often exhibit a fear or shame about eating, excessive cravings, "secret" eating habits, and binge eating. Most people who suffer from food addiction readily admit that they know the potential hazards of consuming excessive amounts of food but have lost the ability to control themselves. As they continue to eat and lose even more control, food becomes an absolute obsession, their very reason for living. An unhealthy preoccupation with body weight and image occurs, and these sufferers become trapped in a cycle of uncontrollable food cravings followed by the distress of what this excess food is doing to their physical appearance.

Anorexia nervosa is a paradoxical food addiction. The hallmark of those suffering from anorexia nervosa is an intense fear of gaining weight, leading to behaviors designed to prevent this from happening. Excessive weighing, measuring of body parts, and use of the mirror to check body size and contours are common obsessions. Self-esteem is completely predicated upon body shape and weight, which makes losing weight a monumental accomplishment and one that anorexics view as a symbol of extraordinary discipline.

Those suffering from bulimia nervosa are binge eaters who then purge or rid themselves of the food they just consumed to prevent weight gain. These individuals are ashamed of their eating behavior and figure rapid consumption of large amounts of food will conceal it from others. People with bulimia nervosa will eat until they're in pain or someone interrupts them. Most of the time sufferers rid themselves of the food through induced vomiting, but they also might choose laxatives, fasting, or excessive exercise to compensate for the bingeing.

Compulsive overeaters share some of the same characteristics as people with bulimia. These people start by using food for purposes other than satisfying their hunger. They eventually become addicted to food and lose control over the amount they eat. Sufferers repeatedly go on uncontrollable binges without controlling their weight, and they see this behavior as normal. Compulsive overeaters are typically moderately to severely obese, and their bingeing episodes often consist of junk food, which is eaten in secrecy and away from the observation of others.

Research has shown that the digestion of food proteins may produce substances that have opiate or narcotic properties that the brain finds to be pleasurable. In fact, some experts have shown that pieces of milk and wheat proteins can actually behave like the body's natural narcotic, endorphins, and send messages to the brain of sheer satisfaction. These substances actually carry information by locating and binding to the brain receptors that ordinarily respond to endorphins.

A fundamental part of food addiction is the series of physiological alterations that occur within the body. Food addicts often report cravings or strong, uncontrollable impulses to eat certain foods. Sweets are most commonly desired, but other categories include milk, bread, cheese, peanuts, fruits, and potato chips. Dealing with these addictions often requires professional counseling and support, as sufferers go through a similar cycle of withdrawal, emotional grieving, and, ultimately, a renewed craving for specific foods. Food addictions are easier and cheaper to support than expensive drug addictions; thus they can be more difficult to resolve, since the supply may never be cut off except for a strong will to abstain from ingesting the foods.

Getting help for these conditions is imperative to one's health. Eating disorders are partly a psychological and partly a physical problem. Risks that attend these conditions include malnutrition, esophagus dysfunction, bone disease, hormonal irregularities, and metabolic imbalances.

CUTTING STRESS TO CUT THE CALORIES

It's a well-accepted fact that most of us live in extremely stressful environments. Gaining an understanding of your environmental and psychological stressors is an important first step in removing them from your life or developing strategies that will help minimize their effect on your behavior. Unfortunately, one way people select consciously and unconsciously to manage their stress is through eating. Many people will, in fact, report that their weight tends to fluctuate with the amount of stress they experience in their lives.

Dieting itself can be a stress-inducing activity, especially when the diet consists of severe food restrictions. A study carried out in London showed that dieters are more likely than nondieters to rely on food in times of emotional anxiety or depression. The researchers divided the female volunteers into three groups; the first was placed on a strict diet, the second followed a rigorous exercise program, and the third served as the control group (volunteers neither exercised or dieted but instead carried on with their typical activities). The groups followed their programs for five weeks before their food intake was assessed as they watched a stressful film. Bowls of different types of sweets and nuts were left beside them, and they were given the freedom to eat as much as they liked. By the end of the movie they found that the women who were part of the dieting group ate far more than the others.

Stress management techniques for those who live in extremely stressful homes or work in high-demand jobs can be just as critical to success as the weight loss program. It's imperative that you have not only a clear insight into those aspects of your life that produce anxiety, but an understanding of the ways in which you typically respond. Certain behavioral modification techniques can teach you to recognize the reflex of grabbing for a sweet when you begin to feel uneasy about a work deadline or an awkward social situation. Many of these techniques work by providing the appropriate amount of feedback, where you get in touch with your stressor and at the same time connect with your inclination to eat food to help soothe yourself.

While reducing stress is an important component in cutting back on unnecessary calories, recognizing your group of comfort foods is equally critical. High-fat, high-sugar, high-calorie foods tend to be the most common stress relievers, which helps explain why indulging in these "junk food" comforts means putting on more pounds. Unfortunately, turning to these foods can throw you into a cycle of even more stress. The more you eat, the more weight you gain, then the more anxious you become about the increasing measurements on your scale. You must find a way to break this vicious cycle, and if it's not by reducing your stress, then at least start by reducing the opportunity you have to consume these weight-packing comfort foods. Remove those chocolate candies from your desk at work and empty the cabinets at home of all those cupcakes and bags of potato chips. Replace them with healthier, low-calorie foods such as carrot sticks, grapes, or wheat crackers. If dealing with a difficult boss or creditors bothering you at home means reaching for food, at least make sure it's low in calories and health promoting.

There are hundreds of relaxation techniques, some more popular than others, but all of them share a common goal of easing the mind-body axis. Whether it's yoga, meditation, or simply sitting on a park bench and watching birds fly from one branch to the next, you must find the activity that allows you to be at peace with yourself and the environment. While it's not possible to run to the park every time you encounter a stressor, it is possible to close your eyes momentarily and visualize those particular activities or situations that you find to be relaxing.

I recently had an experience that, in recalling, seems to melt away the anxiety and tension of whatever situation currently swarms around me. I was playing golf at a beautiful course built along the Atlantic Ocean. I was playing the course for the first time, and my golfing partner kept telling me that there was a hole we were going to play that was "out of this world." I knew we were there when I stood on the tee box and looked at the green some 140 yards away. The green seemed to stand by itself, with wild shrubbery growing around it, and just behind as a backdrop was the Atlantic Ocean and its cresting waves crashing against the shoreline. Even my bogey score wasn't enough to taint the beauty of the scene. Since that golf outing, I find myself thinking about that hole and the Atlantic Ocean roaring quietly behind it. You must find your own moment or image that you can mentally reproduce and visit as often as you need to relax and step away from a stressful situation. Some people find this through some of the meditative exercises such as tai chi chuan or yoga, while others are able to close their eyes wherever they are and block out the world around them and focus on a specific image or idea. Simply breathing deeply and saying the word *one* as you exhale can bring about a sense of calm.

OVERCOMING SETBACKS

Any honest discussion about weight loss should include the topic of setbacks—those minifailures that can send you careening off the road of weight loss or temporarily stunt your progress. Even the most successful of dieters have had their fill of disappointments, failing to reach goals at predetermined times or finding the routine that had been working so well suddenly stopped taking off the weight. There are things that happen in all of our lives—the death of a loved one or a major life disruption like the loss of a job—that can deliver a major jolt to our schedules. There are simply times when other issues become more important than counting calories or weighing yourself at the same time on the same scale. Your mind and program must be flexible enough to accommodate these disruptions, but your willpower must be strong enough to bring you back on course once these issues are resolved.

Acknowledging that there will be setbacks on the course of your journey is not an excuse for failure. Instead, it's a realistic forecast of what lies ahead. Why is the weather the number one reason viewers tune in to the news? Because if it's going to rain, you want to know you're going to need an umbrella. If you accept that there will be setbacks somewhere along the course, you'll be much better equipped mentally to deal with them and not allow them to impede your progress. The dieter who begins a program believing the weight will come off smoothly and consistently is only setting the stage for failure and disappointment.

A common pitfall for dieters is believing that an episode of weakness signals that it's time to simply toss the program away. For example, you've started this program and one afternoon you find yourself at a lunch looking over the irresistible dessert tray of sweets. Unable to control yourself any longer, you take a bite of apple pie. After one bite, you go ahead and finish the rest. Often those who aren't truly prepared to handle this minor setback will convince themselves that they've already cheated, so why not throw away the diet for the rest of the day and start up again tomorrow? That's a mistake that repeated several times can spell disaster for your program compliance and your waistline. Instead, take a moment to reflect on what you've just done and the guiding principles of your weight loss program. Take control and refocus on finishing the day strong, going back to the diet and activity plan.

Daily or weekly journals are important if you're dieting, not only to keep track of the food you've eaten or the amount of exercise performed, but also to list other life issues that you need to address. Recording your setbacks is an important way to acknowledge that you've strayed from your preferred behavior. It also forces you to analyze the cause of this disruption, as you must first think about what has transpired before putting your thoughts to paper. Another advantage of recording your setbacks is that it helps you identify the triggers so that in the future you can avoid them if they seem to be lurking around.

A major part of overcoming these disruptions is your attitude. Thinking positively and confidently about your ability to reach your realistic goals can be your greatest weapon against the temptation to give up. If you approach dieting with a defeatist's attitude, then defeat is exactly what you'll face when you hit that first bump in the road. If, however, your mind is conditioned to expect minor disappointments and your faith remains unwavering, you'll find yourself quickly back on the path to weight loss and increased physical activity.

MONITORING YOUR WEIGHT LOSS

It is crucial that you measure your progress on a weekly rather than a daily basis. Proper weight loss is a slow process, and you are working with your body to adjust to physiological changes. Take a long view and summon the patience to cooperate with your body as you undertake this endeavor.

Weigh yourself on the same day at the same time every week. Your weight will naturally fluctuate by a few pounds depending on how much fluid and food is in your system. Do not be discouraged if your progress can't be charted as a smooth, unbroken decline in your weight.

You may also find it helpful to take your measurements with a tape measure, as this is a more accurate gauge of your progress. Muscle weighs three times more than fat. As you exercise, thus converting fat to muscle, your weight might remain stable while you have actually reduced your overall size.

REMEMBER, what has happened in the past is behind you. You may have tried several diets only to lose weight temporarily and regain it in a matter of months. The difference between those past failures and your future success, however, will be measured by what you've learned and how you plan to incorporate those lessons. It might sound like a broken record, but if you expect to have any shot at making these important changes in your life, you need to give yourself a chance to start fresh. Take advantage of your setbacks and arm yourself with the information that has doomed your past efforts. You're now able to construct a road map to success, and if your mind is also on the right track, victory is certainly within your grasp. Honesty about what lies ahead of you and how difficult it might be to accomplish your goals is the only way to directly confront your weight management problems. The body might be weak at times, but a strong mind can heal the psychological damage and inspire the body's cooperation in regaining its health.

PART TWO

GET A HANDLE
ON THE FACTS

CHAPTER 2

CAUSES OF OBESITY AND OVERWEIGHT

We have become a country of people obsessed with weight and its implications on our health and appearance. At any one time, approximately 25 percent of men and 45 percent of women are trying to lose weight. Obesity and weight loss have created one of the world's largest commercial industries. Americans spend more than $33 billion per year on weight control programs and services, yet a look at the increasing rates of obesity over the last twenty years shows that this huge expenditure is having little, if any, effect on our expanding waistlines.

CAUSES OF OBESITY

Overconsumption of Unhealthy Foods

No one factor has contributed more to the world's expanding girth than the overconsumption of high-calorie foods. In no country is this more apparent than the United States, the home of fast food, refined sugars, and processed goods. Big family dinners where we all sat around the kitchen table and discussed the events of the day are quickly becoming a part of our sentimental past. Eating a meal for most of us means ordering take-out or eating out at restaurants. Of course, this is much more convenient than spending hours in the kitchen preparing a big meal, but it also means that we have less control of how our food is prepared. Restaurants are less concerned with taking an extra fifteen minutes to cook food in a healthy manner and tend to serve larger portions than are healthful.

One of the growing trends has been consuming foods full of "empty" calories. Soda, candy, and desserts are full of refined sugar and fat, high in energy but low in nutritional value. High-calorie foods are acceptable if they contain minerals or vitamins, but convenience foods just offer highly concentrated calories and little in return. The busy nature of our lives has made eating on the run less a fix for hunger and more a way of life. Vending machines are an all-too-simple answer when there's no time for a well-balanced meal. Unfortunately, a bag of chips and a bottle of Coke that take the edge off the hunger pangs also add a substantial amount to your day's calorie load. When you do finally sit down to eat a meal, your body needs to burn off not only these new calories, but the extra calories it's consumed in all of the day's little snacks.

Unhealthy, calorie-rich diets combined with a sedentary lifestyle can wreak havoc on our waistlines. This potent one-two punch is most likely responsible for the dramatic rise of overweight and obese conditions that have been noted over the last few decades. If we were a nation that incorporated a moderate amount of physical activity into our daily lives, then the poor dietary choices we make would be less punishing when we stepped on the scale. The truth, however, is that not only are we eating more calories, but we're also burning fewer of them through physical activity such as walking or exercise. This combination has completely disrupted our energy balance, thus producing a country struggling with weight control. We'll discuss more about physical activity in part 5 of the book, but first it's important to understand the energy equation that guides our weight accumulation and loss.

Our weight is inextricably tied to energy balance. All of the foods we eat, whether it's a piece of gum or a can of soda, contain a certain amount of energy calories that can be made available to the body to carry out all of its functions. Not only do we consume energy in food, but over the course of a day, we also expend a certain amount of energy, whether it's walking down a few flights of stairs or even getting up and down from a chair several times. All of these activities increase the amount of energy we use in a day. In order to maintain your weight, the energy that you put in must equal the energy that you burn up. So let's say you consume 5 units of energy, and burn 5 units of energy, then the net gain is 0. But what happens if you consume 5 units of energy but burn only 3 units? You now have a net *gain* of 2 units. These 2 surplus energy units don't just disappear into thin air; instead, the body must find a place for them. That place, unfortunately, is somewhere in those seventy-five billion fat cells, making them expand and thus adding inches to your waistline.

This energy equation also works when trying to understand what's required to shed those excess pounds. If you consume 5 units of energy, but your daily activities cause you to burn off 7 units, then there's a net *loss* of 2 units. These extra units that are lost typically come from those fat cells, thus helping to reduce your weight. This is why you often hear people say, "I'm counting my calories." What they're counting is the amount of energy they're putting into their body. The mistake that most people make, however, is that they ignore the other half of the equation and don't realize that it's equally important to count the calories, or energy units, they burn off.

Fatty foods are the biggest challenge to maintaining a healthy weight, because they pack the most calories per unit volume than the two other major nutrients. At 9 calories per gram, fats more than double the energy-carrying capacity found in carbohydrates and protein, which each carry 4 calories per gram. Understanding these simple energy facts makes it easier to reason why a diet of fast food—burgers and fries or fried mozzarella sticks—dumps large amounts of energy units into your body.

Sugar consumption has been another cause of our expanding waistlines. Most experts have been tirelessly pointing out that our sugar intake is simply off the charts. According to the U.S. Department of Agriculture (USDA), people consuming 2,000 calories per day shouldn't consume more than ten added teaspoons of sugar per day. However, USDA surveys show that Americans are far exceeding this limit, consuming as many as twenty added teaspoons of sugar. These added sugars are found largely in junk food—sodas, cake, and cookies—but are also contained in healthful foods like juices, low-fat snacks, fruit, and nutrition bars and shakes. They squeeze healthier, less calorie-rich foods out of the diet.

In the year 1977–1978, the government found that sugars constituted only 11 percent of the average person's calories. Now, this number has ballooned to 16 percent for the average American adult and as much as 20 percent for American teenagers. Soft drinks are largely responsible for these increases, containing approximately nine teaspoons of added sugar in a single twelve-ounce can. In fact, the per-household consumption of soda has doubled since 1974, something not particularly surprising since the American Medical Association expressed concerns about these foods and beverages back in 1942. Because sugar has little nutritional value and can trigger food cravings, reducing the amount of sugar calories in our diets is an important and effective way to prevent unwanted weight gain. However, the enthusiasm with which many gimmick diets promote weight loss based strictly on reducing carbohydrates is overstating the case. Reducing carbohydrate consumption to near normal levels is part of the solution, but it's certainly not the complete answer.

A Sedentary Life

Each year a new survey shows how physically inactive we're becoming. Most of these changes started in the 1980s, but the 1990s will forever be remembered as a decade of convenience. This energy wouldn't be such a bad thing if the body had a demand that equaled it. The increasing popularity of sedentary forms of entertainment, like watching TV, spending time on computers, and watching videos at home, along with the convenience of modern transportation (cars, buses, and subways), have led to a dramatic decline in our level of physical activity and thus a lower demand for energy. Delivery service has become less a privilege used by those willing to pay a few extra dollars and more a routine and expected service.

According to the National Health and Nutrition Examination Survey, 24 percent of American adults are completely sedentary, and 54 percent spend inadequate time in physical activity. Four in ten U.S. adults say that they never engage in any exercises, sports, or physically active hobbies in their leisure time. Sedentary behavior has been identified as a risk factor for a variety of chronic health conditions, including coronary heart disease, high blood pressure, colon cancer, and diabetes.

It's no mere coincidence that the President's Council on Exercise and the Surgeon General's Office have led campaigns to increase our level of exercise. Not only is this exercise beneficial in keeping our weight from ballooning, but it's extremely important in maintaining the health of many of our organs, including the heart and its network of blood vessels that course throughout the body. The American Heart Association and many other health professional organizations recommend a weekly schedule of physical activity—a minimum of thirty minutes a day for three to five days a week. Weight-bearing exercises and increasing your heart rate are two aspects of physical activity that show the most benefit in preventing heart disease and osteoporosis, the bone-thinning disease.

Physical activity is the one aspect of energy expenditure over which we have the most control. Our metabolism and the energy of food digestion are expenditures that are determined mostly by physics and genetics. If consumption of calories outpaces energy expenditure, weight gain is inevitable. Thus our decreasing level of physical activity forces the body to store the excess calories as fat. Studies repeatedly show that by making a modest commitment to an exercise program or by participating in more leisurely activities that require energy expenditure, people can do a lot to reverse unwanted weight gain and prevent more pounds from accumulating. The role of physical activity and weight loss is discussed at length in chapter 10.

Emotional Eating

The primary purpose of food, for our ancestors, was sustenance. Killing animals and harvesting crops were simply the means of providing the energy needed to live. Many anthropologists who discuss the physical appearance of early man often note that his body habitus was quite different from ours—more lean and flexible, made to live in more natural surroundings and carry out the strenuous daily activities of life. What is not well documented is whether early man had the emotional relationships to food that many have today, relationships that contribute to eating patterns that promote weight gain and obesity.

Our body has a complex system of hunger, appetite, and satisfaction (satiety) that's mediated by a network of nerves and chemical messengers. We receive impulses to eat as well as impulses to stop eating. Most of this is involuntary and happens without us thinking about it, but there are times when we override these signals, eating what we want whenever we want. In these instances, food is no longer just our source of fuel; it carries an additional meaning that has less to do with satisfying hunger signals than with fulfilling an emotional or psychological void.

People who are either clinically depressed or experience bouts of depressed mood will often discuss how they notice a cycle of weight gain and loss that correlates directly with their emotional state. Some of this weight gain is attributed to a decrease in physical activity, but much of it is a result of overeating, particularly calorie-dense foods such as chocolate or fried foods. Food consumption is triggered not just by hunger, but by feelings of angst, sadness, or guilt. It's believed that food releases certain chemicals in the brain called endorphins, which mediate a feeling of happiness. Depressed people can enter a cycle of excess consumption where food helps to alleviate the bad feelings, so the worse a person feels, the more food he or she is willing to consume. These "comfort" foods tend to be the more unhealthy, high-calorie variety.

Rich, high-calorie foods have also taken on significance in our idea of celebration. The most memorable events you've attended probably included an abundance of fine food. At such events, even those who claim to be on strict diets usually cast aside their self-imposed limitations and join the fray. The rationalization is simple: Celebrations happen only occasionally, so why not indulge for the one afternoon or evening? Admittedly, there is something delightful about discarding one's concerns. In truth, a rare afternoon or evening of overindulgence will not do any lasting damage. The danger mounts, however, if this attitude begins to justify excess on a regular basis.

Genetics

There are people who never seem to gain an ounce of weight regardless of how much or what they eat. Others seem only to have to look at a dessert menu and the pounds start piling on. Certainly, various levels of physical activity partly account for this difference, but the tiny genes buried in our cells that we inherit from our parents are the most powerful factor. One need only look at cases of familial obesity to witness the effects of genetic predisposition. Studies show that if a person has one obese parent, he or she has a 60 percent chance of becoming obese. If both your parents are obese, the chances jump to 90 percent.

Researchers have examined the weight patterns of adopted children to further establish the link between genetics and obesity. After comparing the weights of the adopted children to those of their biological parents and adopted parents, most children were found to be similar to their biological parents in weight. Twin studies also help highlight the role genetics plays in our weight patterns. Even when raised in separate environments, identical twins who share *exactly* the same genes are twice as likely as fraternal twins who share *some* genes to weigh the same.

The understanding of our genetics, otherwise known as DNA or the blueprint of life, has been one of the greatest scientific achievements recorded in our time. Our knowledge of genes has increased exponentially over the last couple of decades, but there's still a tremendous amount of information that we don't know. With the recent mapping of the entire human genome, scientists will hopefully be able to identify all of the genes responsible for life's functions, whether it's understanding our body's metabolism or why our hearts typically beat in a rhythmic fashion.

I've often heard people who've battled weight control problems all of their lives complain that they've done everything they can, but being overweight is simply in their genes. For some, this statement might be partially correct, but the explanation behind it can be quite complicated. Our genes determine everything from the color of our hair and our height to where our body will deposit excess weight. Some of us are born with genes that make it easier for us to gain weight, but whether or not we are overweight is entirely within our control.

Many people with an inherited propensity to gain weight throw up their hands and resign themselves to a life of obesity, to their own hurt. The good news is that your level of physical activity and the diet you consume can overcome your genetic tendencies to gain extra weight. You may be born to gain weight, but you can live to prevent it from happening. If you're empowered with the knowledge that the numbers showing up on your scale can largely be controlled by behavioral modifications, then you're at least giving yourself a fighting chance.

One of the most recent areas of obesity research has been on the gene that codes for leptin, a hormone believed to be important in suppressing appetite. Researchers believe that leptin also increases energy expenditure, influences the fat cells to store less fat, and triggers some to self-destruct. Leptin is further believed to have other regulatory roles in the body, such as stimulating the growth of new blood vessels, acting on the bone marrow cells to enhance their maturation into specialized cells, promoting the formation of red blood cells, and helping to support a normal immune system.

Most of the work with leptin has been done on mice and the discovery of the obesity gene, *ob*. Mice with a defective *ob* gene fail to produce leptin even when they're grossly overweight and can eventually gain in size three times that of a normal mouse. You might ask, if leptin is such a powerful appetite suppressant and important component of weight control, why not simply inject it into overweight people? The simple answer is that overweight people don't lack sufficient amounts of leptin; in fact, studies of their blood samples show that they have elevated levels. What researchers believe is that as fat increases and leptin rises, the leptin receptors in the brain become less responsive, thus diminishing leptin's effects.

MEDICAL CONDITIONS
Thyroid

There are a few medical conditions that trigger obesity, and these conditions are treatable once diagnosed. There is one gland that has consistently demonstrated its influence on our body's weight. The thyroid gland, located just beneath the voice box, is responsible for producing thyroid hormones. While these hormones are responsible for all types of bodily functions, the one most relevant to our discussion is metabolism.

If the thyroid gland becomes underactive and doesn't produce enough thyroid hormone, or if the hormone that is produced turns out to be defective, then this condition is categorized as hypothyroidism. If you have hypothyroidism, a complex set of interactions occurs that results in lowering your metabolism. Thus, the line of thinking goes like this: Decreased functional thyroid hormone leads to a lowered metabolism, which causes a decrease in the amount of energy burned, resulting in weight gain. Even with this chain of events, however, most people who have hypothyroidism don't see the dramatic type of weight gain that tips their scale into the overweight or obese categories. Someone must have hypothyroidism for a prolonged period of time before it results in increased body weight. Also, hypothyroidism is a very treatable medical condition, and a daily course of synthetic thyroid pills has been most effective in bringing thyroid hormone levels in the blood back to normal.

Symptoms of hypothyroidism can often be confused with other illnesses. Common signs include hair loss, constipation, unexplained weight gain, mental sluggishness, intolerance to cold temperatures, dry, rough skin, and excessive fatigue.

Cushing's Disease

A rare cause of obesity is a condition called Cushing's disease, which develops when the diminutive adrenal glands secrete too many hormones. One of these hormones, cortisol, can produce distinct physical characteristics when found in excessive amounts. A person can have increased body weight, particularly obesity in the stomach and chest area, swollen extremities, excessive hair growth, purplish lines in the skin that stretch along the abdomen, and bluish areas that look like bruises. Beyond the physical symptoms, however, patients can also experience weakness and fatigue, high blood pressure, personality changes, increased urination frequency, and for women a loss of their period. Cushing's patients have quite a typical appearance, with chubby, rounded cheeks, noticeable fatty areas in the neck or just above the collarbone, and a predominance of abdominal obesity.

Cushing's disease is diagnosed through a combination of laboratory and physical findings. Blood tests will reveal increased steroid production and the failure of the body to stop making steroids when given the stimulus to stop. Doctors combine these laboratory findings with characteristic physical signs in the patient in order to make a diagnosis.

Insulinoma

An insulinoma is a rare tumor located in the pancreas, which over-secretes the hormone insulin. It most commonly appears in people between the ages of fifty and seventy, but it can occur at any age. This hyperproduction of insulin causes a major disruption of the typically regulated insulin levels and leads to a condition of hypoglycemia, in which the glucose supply in the blood is greatly diminished. The hormone insulin is important because it works to help the cells absorb glucose, our body's major source of energy. When we eat a meal, the pancreas is stimulated to secrete insulin into the blood; this insulin travels throughout the body and promotes the absorption of glucose by the many cells that use its energy. Because the sugar levels are continuously depleted, patients will automatically increase their caloric intake to fill the perceived energy void. This increased consumption can lead to obesity in some, but most patients with insulinomas aren't obese.

Patients are tested for this condition by entering a seventy-two-hour fasting state in which they're not allowed to eat anything that might increase their blood sugar levels. After this seventy-two-hour period, blood tests are taken to measure the level of sugar in the blood. Most patients with insulinomas will demonstrate markedly decreased blood sugar levels within twenty-four hours, while others may require more time.

Once the diagnosis has been made, acute treatment involves intravenous infusion of glucose. Oral medications can also be administered to help raise the blood sugar level, but their effects may last only a short time. Surgery remains the definitive therapy: the portion of the pancreas that contains the insulinoma will be resected.

MEDICATIONS

Steroids

When most of us think of steroids, we think of weight lifters or athletes with gigantic muscles bulging out of the seams of their shirts and trousers. This is because anabolic steroids have for a long time been popular with athletes trying to gain bulk and strength for their respective sports. There is, however, a medicinal variety of steroids commonly used for a variety of medical conditions, including autoimmune disorders (such as lupus) and severe asthma.

Similar to the anabolic steroids, these medicinal steroids are quite effective at carrying out their primary goals, but they also have their fair share of side effects. The one most relevant to our discussion is increased weight. People who are either on steroids for a long period of time or are on heavy doses have a much greater likelihood of gaining weight, typically in the face or abdomen. Often a puffy face or increased fatty hump at the base of the neck are signs that the person might be taking steroids. Unfortunately, many people who are on steroids need them to combat their severe medical condition, so in these cases, the side effect of weight gain is much preferred to the underlying medical problem, which is often life-threatening.

Tricyclic Antidepressants

This family of medications has revolutionized the treatment of depression and in some cases alleviated physical pain. However, one of the common side effects is weight gain, something that should be explained to all patients before they begin therapy. As with the medicinal steroids just mentioned, patients and their doctors must consider the pros and cons of antidepressant therapy in determining whether the medication's potential benefit is great enough to risk a weight gain. This decision is an individual one that should be made after an informed conversation between patient and doctor. It's important, however, to remember that tricyclic antidepressants, while often effective at alleviating depressed mood, aren't the only treatment option available. Other medications have been shown to be equally effective, as have behavioral modification techniques, which, instead of working through this chemical pathway, harness mental power.

CHAPTER 3

IF THIS DOESN'T SCARE YOU, NOTHING WILL

Health Concerns of Overweight and Improper Dieting

America has a major public health problem that's triggering diseases and deaths that are far too preventable—overweight/obesity. Every week another study splashes into the headlines, highlighting the increasing girth of our country and the rising incidence of medical conditions that accompany it. The statistics tell most of the story: 97.1 million Americans over the age of twenty are overweight, an astounding 55 percent of our adult population; 59.4 percent of men and 46.9 percent of women over twenty years of age are battling their bulging waistlines. Most alarming are the number of children who find themselves outside the range of normal weight: 14 percent of children between the ages of six and eleven are overweight, while 11 percent of adolescents between the ages of twelve and seventeen are struggling to keep their weight within a range considered to be healthy.

Obesity, a more severe measure of overweight, is of greater concern because it refers specifically to having an abnormally high proportion of body fat. Studies have shown that while being overweight can predispose a person to medical problems such as heart disease, diabetes, and high blood pressure, obesity increases the risk for these conditions dramatically. Nearly a quarter of U.S. adults are obese, and less than half actually maintain a weight that's considered to be healthy. If you don't believe the statistics from the National Institutes of Health, simply conduct a survey yourself. Go to an area full of pedestrian traffic and pick a corner or specific point to count the people as they pass by. Just on visual inspection alone, count the first twenty people who randomly walk by and categorize them as normal or overweight. You'll soon find that the prevalence of overweight people is as disappointing as the statistics demonstrate.

Smoking-related illnesses kill approximately four hundred thousand people each year, followed closely by the three hundred thousand deaths believed to be related to obesity. The costs, beyond the physical sacrifices, are enormous. The United States spends $99.2 billion each year on costs attributed to medications, hospitalizations, or doctors' visits; 39.3 million workdays are lost related to obesity, and 62.7 million physicians' office visits are made each year to address obesity-related medical problems.

Anyone who's trying to gain control of his or her weight must first be armed with knowledge of the enemy. Obesity is becoming a worldwide epidemic, particularly here in the United States, where 55 percent of adults are overweight. If it were simply an issue of how one looked in a bathing suit, then most doctors and public health advocates wouldn't be ringing the alarm so loudly. Instead, being overweight or obese leads to myriad health problems, many of which can be reversed or improved by bringing one's weight back into a normal range.

While you might want to fit into a dress that's become too tight or a suit with trousers that are difficult to button, the imperative to lose weight goes way beyond what you see in the mirror. Obesity causes most of its damage quietly, wreaking havoc on the body's internal organs, most notably the heart and its network of blood vessels. For many people suffering from severe obesity, losing weight isn't an issue of shopping for beach bikinis; it's a matter of the quality of life and avoiding an unnecessary death.

Many obese patients who have been in my care have been subjected to a tremendous amount of suffering, whether it's from diabetes, joint arthritis, or musculoskeletal pain. Their bodies are often racked with pain, and simple activities such as tying one's shoes or bending down to pick up items become a major effort. Even physicians often feel helpless as these good people try repeatedly without success to reverse the weight gain that has cost them jobs and relationships and made them targets of societal ridicule.

Carrying extra weight for a long period of time ages the body much faster and more strenuously than normal. Fatigue sets in quicker, and physical endurance is dramatically reduced to the point that walking up one flight of stairs requires a brief rest before being able to move on. X-rays of the spines and knees of these patients tell the story of a lifetime of unrelenting pounding, with joints eroded and the ends of the bones scarred from arthritic changes. For many, embarrassment sets in when the excess weight becomes so unmanageable, it's difficult to maintain adequate self-hygiene. I'll never forget a patient I was treating during a rotation through the emergency room. After walking into the room, introducing myself, and recording her medical history, I told her I was going to examine her, and she burst into tears. "I'm sorry for not being clean," she sobbed. "It's difficult for me to get around and do the things a woman is supposed to do."

A large part of losing weight and maintaining a healthy weight is first establishing a substantive purpose for the weight loss that will inspire long-term loss instead of a temporary drop. I often hear people say, "I must lose ten pounds in a couple of weeks, because I'm going to a wedding." Some of them might actually lose those ten pounds and feel good at the wedding, but in most cases, as soon as the bride and groom are off on their honeymoon, those pounds begin to creep right back on. This short course of weight loss tied to a discrete event is nothing more than temporary happiness and a setup for permanent disaster. These people are constantly on and off diets, losing weight based on their next event.

Those who tend to lose weight and keep it off are people who say, "I need to lose this extra weight to improve the quality of my life." These people have not only identified their problem, they've also acknowledged the larger implications of being overweight or obese—the potential for a lifetime of medical complications and an overall sense of sickness. Committing yourself to weight loss because it makes sense in the big picture of your health and your interaction with the environment is the psychological starting point that can be critical in helping you stay focused on keeping your weight under control.

WHERE FAT ACCUMULATES MAKES A DIFFERENCE IN YOUR HEALTH

Most people want to lose certain pockets of fat that won't go away. Whether under the arms, between the legs, or at the sides of the abdomen ("love handles"), fat tends to accumulate differently in all of us, as if it has a mind of its own. People who have lost and gained weight a few times can predict with great accuracy the area of the body that will change.

Experts aren't sure how fat is programmed to deposit and shed in certain places, but some of it is likely due to genetics. Others have suggested certain exercises can get rid of fat in targeted areas, but the results of these studies are debatable at best. The important thing to understand is that where fat accumulates on your body could have a major impact on your risk for disease. Some people store fat in the upper body region. In overweight people, this particular distribution is called android, or "apple-shaped," obesity. This type of fat distribution is more common in men and is recognizable by a potbelly with small buttocks and thighs—like an apple on a stick. Alcohol intake and high testosterone levels are believed to encourage this fat pattern. Researchers have found that android obesity is associated with a greater risk for heart disease, high blood pressure, and type II diabetes. Other fat cells typically empty fat directly into the circulation, but in these people the content of abdominal fat cells is sent straight to the liver. This can interfere with the liver's normal functioning, altering protein metabolism and reducing the liver's ability to break down insulin that's no longer needed.

Most women store fat in the lower body region. This is called gynecoid, or "pear-shaped," obesity and is indicated by a smaller abdomen but much larger buttocks and thighs. It's believed that the female hormones estrogen and progesterone play a key role in this fat distribution pattern, a theory that is strengthened by the fact that women tend to switch over to the upper obesity shape once they drastically diminish the production of these hormones after menopause. The pear shape distribution is associated with fewer health risks, but if women are twenty pounds more obese than men with potbellies, they begin to suffer similar risks. Regardless of what type of fat distribution pattern you have, remember that any excess fat poses its own health dangers.

HEART DISEASE

Half a million Americans will lose their lives this year to heart disease, making it the number one killer in America. Obesity has been shown to be one of the biggest risk factors for cardiovascular disease, largely because it triggers so many other medical conditions that directly and indirectly lead to heart-related conditions. High cholesterol levels, long believed to be a risk factor in the formation of atherosclerosis, or plaque buildup in blood vessels, have been shown in several studies to be associated with overweight, obesity, and weight gain. It's not just how much extra fat you're carrying, but exactly where that fat is stored that can have greater health implications. Fat location makes a difference, as researchers have found higher total cholesterol levels in people whose obesity is predominantly in the abdomen and who measure an increased waist-to-hip circumference ratio.

Other circulating blood particles are elevated in people with even the slightest weight gains. Triglycerides, the major storage form of fat, and a factor that increases the risk for heart disease, are directly linked to a person's level of obesity. Studies looking at all ages and gender have demonstrated that the higher the body mass index (BMI), the higher the level of triglycerides, and thus the greater the risk for heart disease. (BMI is explained in chapter 7.)

Coronary arteries, the blood vessels that actually nourish the heart muscle, can also suffer from disease as a result of obesity. Research continues to show that the higher the BMI level, the greater the risk for disease. According to the Mayo Clinic, weight gains of as little as ten to twenty pounds can increase coronary artery disease risk by 25 percent. Weight gains of approximately forty-five or more pounds can increase the risk for coronary heart disease by as much as 250 percent.

HYPERTENSION

The blood pressure we measure with a stethoscope ... amount of pressure our blood exerts against the wall... sels. This recording is an important measure because the amount of work the heart is performing and the co....... of the blood vessels that carry blood and its nourishment throughout the body. Blood pressure is recorded as two numbers—the systolic pressure (upper number) over the diastolic pressure (lower number). The systolic pressure is the force of blood in the arteries as the heart beats. The diastolic pressure is the force of blood in the arteries as the heart relaxes between beats.

High blood pressure, or hypertension, is a condition in which a person has a consistent blood pressure reading of 140/90. Fifty million Americans have high blood pressure, roughly one in five adults. Approximately forty-four thousand people die each year as a direct result of their high blood pressure, and hypertension is believed to play some role in more than two hundred thousand deaths. Elevated blood pressure delivers most of its damage on the heart and arteries, mostly because it causes the heart to work harder than normal. This increases the risk of heart attack, stroke, kidney failure, and damage to the eyes. Once arteries become scarred, hardened, and less flexible, they aren't able to supply the amount of blood the body's organs need. If the body's organs don't get enough oxygen and nutrients, they can't work properly and can decline into failure.

Overweight conditions and obesity have been shown to be critical risk factors for developing high blood pressure. In fact, data from the NHANES III study has shown that the prevalence of high blood pressure increases progressively with higher levels of BMI in men and women. Hypertension is believed to be six times more likely to affect obese adults than people of average weight. Of all the overweight- and obesity-related health conditions, researchers have found that high blood pressure is the most common for both men and women. Several studies have confirmed what doctors have suspected for a long time— obese individuals (BMI of 30 or more) are twice as likely to develop high blood pressure as their normal-weight counterparts (BMI of 18.5 to 24.9).

In a large international study of salt (Intersalt) that involved ten thousand men and women, researchers found that a twenty-two-pound-higher body weight is associated with an increase of the systolic pressure by 3.0 mm Hg (millimeters of mercury) and an increase of the diastolic pressure by 2.3 mm Hg. These slight differences alone translate into an estimated 12 percent increased risk for coronary heart disease and a 24 percent increased risk for stroke.

How does obesity lead to increased blood pressure? Scientists are still working out all of the details, but they do have some answers that can help explain what goes wrong. Obesity is believed to cause increased levels of insulin, which in turn cause the kidneys to retain sodium (like that in salt). This salt retention leads to an increase in the volume of fluid in our blood vessels, thus increasing the amount of pressure exerted against the artery walls and leading to high blood pressure.

The good news, however, is that weight loss can be important in significantly reducing high blood pressure. Our blood vessels become more flexible, the total blood volume decreases, and a particular kidney pathway is suppressed—all leading to a reduction in blood pressure.

DIABETES

There are two major types of diabetes—type I and type II. Type I, also called juvenile diabetes, typically occurs in childhood and has more to do with a genetic defect that leads to poor insulin hormone production than it does with lifestyle behaviors. Type II, however, accounts for as many as 95 percent of diabetics cases, and while there is some component of genetic error, numerous studies and clinical evidence have shown us that lifestyle choices greatly influence the presence and outcome of this disease.

Type II diabetes is a major cause of death, heart disease, kidney disease, stroke, blindness, blood vessel disease, and limb amputation. We now know that not all, but most, type II diabetics are overweight. The development of type II diabetes has been found to be associated with weight gain after age eighteen in both men and women. In fact, some studies have shown that approximately a quarter of all new cases of adult diabetes are due to a weight gain of eleven pounds or more. For those wondering how your BMI correlates with your risk for diabetes, try this—for each additional unit of BMI over twenty-two, the relative risk of diabetes increases by 25 percent.

The encouraging news, however, is that simple lifestyle changes for type II diabetics can bring on dramatic health improvements without medication. See the section on diabetes in chapter 10 for more information on this subject.

NEGATIVE PSYCHOSOCIAL EFFECTS

It's not easy being overweight in a critical society that places so much value on physical appearance. Many of my patients who were large even as children have often described this aspect of their lives as a living nightmare. Messages are constantly broadcast, whether in the popular media or in the way others judge us, that women should be thin and fit and that being overweight is nothing more than a manifestation of a lack of self-control. We form negative attitudes toward overweight people in our childhood, labeling them with condescending names and purposely excluding them from our social circles. The social isolation of a young child can seriously scar the mind and lead one to a life of depressed mood and feelings of being a societal misfit. Discrimination starts out as not being picked for a team during school recess and leads to unfair bias in employment opportunities, college acceptance, job earnings, and marital opportunities.

People who are overweight often experience a tremendous amount of anxiety and stress. Not only are they forced to deal with disapproving stares, finger-pointing, and whispering, but they are also constantly reminded that they are unacceptable. This relentless feeling of being scrutinized or ridiculed can place an enormous amount of mental stress on a person, so much at times that some people begin to question their self-worth and, in the most severe cases, even their right to live. Stress is one of those factors that can actually cause the weight gain on the one hand and be the result of this gain on the other. Food for many becomes a source of comfort, filling an emotional void and helping people deal with a vast array of psychological issues that seem to be driving them further into a cycle of depression and isolation.

GALLBLADDER

The gallbladder is a small organ nestled into the right upper quadrant of your abdomen. It carries out several functions, including the production and secretion of bile, which helps digest fatty foods. The gallbladder is typically a quiet organ, living most of its life anonymously, helping us digest the fats of french fries and pie crusts. However, if you've ever had a gallstone, this tiny organ takes on mammoth significance as you experience intense abdominal cramping pain.

Many factors are associated with gallstone formation, but overweight and obesity tend to be two of the most critical. Scientists aren't exactly sure how being overweight leads directly to gallbladder disease, but what they do know is that your risk for gallbladder problems increases as your weight increases. Some studies have shown that when a woman's BMI is above 40, her risk for either gallstones or the surgery required to remove them is as high as twenty per one thousand women per year. This is more than six times greater than women with a BMI of less than 24, where only three per one thousand women are affected. While women tend to be at a greater risk for gallstones, men are also affected, and studies looking at weight gain in men show a similar, though less drastic, increase in risk.

It stands to reason that weight loss will reduce your risk for gallbladder disease, but there's a caveat you need to be made aware of. Weight loss itself, especially rapid weight loss or a large amount of weight, can actually increase your chances of developing gallstones. This doesn't mean you shouldn't lose weight, but you should understand that a slow, gradual weight loss of one to two pounds a week is less likely to cause gallstones.

OBSTRUCTIVE SLEEP APNEA

Apnea simply means a temporary absence of breathing. Obstructive sleep apnea is a serious medical condition in which a person stops breathing for short periods during sleep. These people are also more prone to snoring, as the soft tissue in the back of the throat vibrates during the breathing cycle, thus producing the noise of snoring. It's no mere coincidence that overweight people tend to snore more often and suffer from daytime sleepiness.

When the upper airway is blocked during sleep, the person breaks the sleep cycle and awakens—not to the level of consciousness as if completely awake, but enough to disrupt continuous sleep; thus the body doesn't feel it's had a complete night's sleep. Most people with sleep apnea have a BMI of 30 or greater, and scientists have found that the severity of sleep apnea is related to the degree of obesity.

Large neck girth in both men and women who snore is highly predictive of sleep apnea. Researchers have found that men with a neck circumference of seventeen inches or greater and women whose neck circumference is sixteen inches or greater are at higher risk for sleep apnea. This, of course, should be taken in context and with the understanding that some people such as weight lifters or athletes have larger neck sizes due to increased muscular development in and around the neck. It's unlikely that they suffer the same increased risk as someone whose neck size results from increased fat tissue.

Beyond snoring and sleep disruption, it's also important to note that obstructive sleep apnea can increase your risk for congestive heart failure. This makes weight loss even more important. Some studies have demonstrated that by losing as little as 10 percent of your body weight, you can reduce the severity of sleep apnea by 50 percent.

OSTEOARTHRITIS

Osteoarthritis is a common joint disorder believed to affect as many as eight million Americans. It most commonly strikes the knees, hips, and lower back. Unlike rheumatoid arthritis, which appears to be an immune system–mediated disease, osteoarthritis appears to be a disease of wear and tear on the joint structures, most notably the cartilage that cushions the end of the upper bone (femur) and lower bone (tibia). Doctors believe that excessive pressure on the joints leads to a gradual erosion of the cartilage cushion, resulting in the bones of the upper and lower legs grinding against one another and leading to deformity and extreme pain. In more severe cases of the disease, sufferers require a total joint replacement surgery, where surgeons take out the natural joint and replace it with a synthetic one.

It only makes sense that the heavier you are for prolonged periods of time, the greater your risk for developing osteoarthritis. Studies have not only shown this to be the case, but they've all confirmed that women stand at a greater risk for developing osteoarthritis than men at the same level of weight gain.

When I'm visited by an overweight or obese patient who complains of joint pain and whose X-rays show early evidence of osteoarthritis, one of the first things I do is advise that patient to get rid of some of the excess weight. People who suffer from osteoarthritis and joint pain can enter a vicious cycle: the joint pain makes physical activity too painful, so they adopt a more sedentary lifestyle. This, of course, means a more fertile ground for developing obesity. Losing weight is critical, as confirmed by one study that showed a decrease in BMI of 2 units or more during a ten-year period decreased the odds for developing knee osteoarthritis by more than 50 percent. Other studies have shown that those patients with osteoarthritis who lose weight tend to experience an improvement in their pain during movement of the knee joint and require less pain-relieving medication.

CANCER

Cancer is the second leading cause of death in the United States, following heart disease, which is the number one killer. There are so many types of cancer that can affect any organ or tissue in the body that it's difficult to make a generalization about the relationship between obesity and cancer. While scientists continue to search for clues that might lead to a cure and better treatment, prevention remains key. Several studies have shown that certain cancers, while not necessarily caused directly by obesity, show an association with overweight.

Colon Cancer

More researchers are pointing to a potentially positive relation between obesity and colon cancer in men, but a weaker association in women. However, recent studies such as the Nurses' Health Study, in which more than one hundred thousand nurses are regularly followed, suggest that the relationship between colon cancer and obesity in women may be more similar to that seen in men than first thought. In men, obesity seems to be a greater predictive risk factor for distal colon cancer, which also includes the rectum. Something else to consider is the waist-to-hip ratio. The higher this relationship, even in leaner women, the greater the association with significantly increased risk of colon polyps.

Breast Cancer

The relationship between obesity and the development of breast cancer is a murky one. Several studies have shown that obesity is directly related to breast cancer deaths mostly in postmenopausal women, most significantly ten or more years after menopause. However, in those women who haven't yet passed through menopause, oddly enough, obesity appears to be associated with a decrease in breast cancer–related deaths. Circulating estrogens have been linked to an increased risk for breast cancer, but postmenopausal women experience a significant drop in estrogen due to the hormonal changes of menopause. So where is the estrogen coming from? Peripheral fat is the primary source of these estrogens, thus adding to the risk for breast cancer.

It is difficult to precisely advise women with this complicated pre- and postmenopausal relationship between obesity and breast cancer. Nonetheless, understanding that a gain of more than twenty pounds from age eighteen to midlife doubles a woman's risk for breast cancer tips the scales in favor of recommending weight loss.

Endometrial Cancer

Obesity has long been considered a risk factor for endometrial cancer, or cancer of the uterine lining. According to a report on obesity issued by the National Institutes of Health, obese women with a BMI of 30 or greater increase their risk for endometrial cancer to three times that of normal-weight women.

YO-YO DIETING

If I had a nickel for every time I heard someone utter, "No thanks, I'm on a diet," I'd be somewhere on the *Forbes* list of the five hundred wealthiest Americans. So many people are on or have been on diets that it seems like a rite of passage for most women and men who find their trousers much tighter than they were a year ago. Unfortunately, dieting has become a trend—in a strange way, a hip culture that allows people to rifle off the specifics of their diet and all of the weight loss results that they've been promised. What most people don't realize is that 90–95 percent of people who go on a diet fail for some reason, but many of these high-profile gimmick diets don't want to address that.

The consequences of yo-yo dieting were first observed by researcher Kelly Brownell of Yale University. Using rats, he examined the effects of repeated cycles of weight loss and regain. He found that not only did it take the rats longer to lose the weight on subsequent cycles, but they also gained it back faster the more they cycled. First, the rats were put on a calorie-restricted diet. After a certain period of time, they were refed. During the second cycle of restriction, the rats needed a total of forty-six days to lose the weight that had taken them only twenty-one days previously. It was also easier for future weight gain. It took the rats only fourteen days on the second off-cycle to regain the same amount of weight that had taken them forty-six days to gain previously.

There are no completed studies yet in humans to confirm this yo-yo effect, but athletes will paint a similar picture if you ask them about their course of weight loss and weight gain between seasons. Typically, the off-season is a period of weight gain for athletes as they reduce the number of hours that they spend working out and increase the amount of food they consume throughout the day. Just before the season starts, athletes return to a preseason training camp, where they are put through long, strenuous workouts and their weight is closely monitored by the team's trainers. It's during this period that a lot of the weight gained during the off-season is actually lost. But the more veteran athletes will be quick to tell you that each progressive year it becomes more difficult to lose the weight that they had before the start of the last season.

The overall goal of losing weight remains an important health measure, especially for those who are considered to be obese. However, it's also important to find a program of healthy weight loss that will help you shed the excess pounds slowly and through techniques or behavioral changes that can last a lifetime. What many people don't know, unfortunately, is that constant weight fluctuations carry their own hidden health dangers.

One concern about this weight cycling is the alteration in cholesterol levels. A study in the *Journal of the American College of Cardiology* found that women who lost at least ten pounds three or more times had an average 7 percent lower HDL (good) cholesterol than women who maintained a stable weight. This is significant because low levels of HDL cholesterol have been associated with a greater chance of heart disease.

Recent studies, including the Framingham Heart Study, the Multiple Risk Factor Intervention Trial, and the Harvard Alumni Study, have shown that these fluctuations in body weight have been associated with adverse health effects, including death from all causes and coronary heart disease in both men and women. The studies found that it didn't matter if your trend was to gain or lose weight, if you experienced these cycles often or greatly, the result was a higher risk of health problems. In fact, the Harvard study showed that continuous weight changes increased the rates of death by over 50 percent when compared with rates for weight-stable individuals.

These potential dangers of yo-yo dieting are not meant to discourage weight loss, as most experts will agree that the health risks of being overweight or obese are proven and outweigh the potential complications one might find while weight cycling. The suggestion that chronic dieting makes future weight loss even more difficult and potentially leads to metabolic derangement makes it all the more important for dieters to think carefully about the program they ultimately choose to join. Diets promising rapid weight loss through a gimmick eating scheme or with a pill that will burn fat are only a setup for future failure. Not only are there serious health implications, the psychological disappointment from repeated weight loss failures could seriously erase the mental edge that's needed to persevere when the chips are down.

STARVATION DIETS

It doesn't take much in the way of scientific knowledge to know that if you don't eat food and still perform some of the activities of daily living, you're bound to lose weight. In fact, many of the early diets severely restricted calorie consumption, in essence putting dieters through a period of starvation. I've seen the effects of this type of diet in one of my cousins, and his weight loss was so dramatic that people wondered if he had taken sick. All of his life he had battled his weight, chronically on and off diets, losing and gaining weight almost as often as the change of seasons. In a matter of a few months, he had lost eighty or more pounds, so much weight that he had to purchase a new wardrobe. I remember him swearing that this was the last diet he would ever need, because this time he was going to keep the weight off for good. Everyone, of course, wanted to know his secret, and surprisingly, it wasn't one of those popular fad diets of the time. Instead, he had simply stopped eating and answered his hunger with large volumes of water, drinking as much as a gallon a day. When, however, he did have an uncontrollable urge to eat, he stayed away from fried, heavy foods, instead eating a plate of fruits or vegetables.

He kept the weight off for at least half the year, but a diet of water and occasional fruits and vegetables was too difficult to maintain. Slowly his food choices returned to starches and meats, and slowly the weight came creeping back. The only negative consequence of his diet seemed to be that once again he had met another dieting failure; but what none of us knew at the time was that he was putting his health at great jeopardy. While weight can be lost through these severe calorie-restricted diets, they pose tremendous health risks. Fat is the first to be attacked, as the body breaks it down to yield some of the energy that it has stored. Unfortunately, the body also begins breaking down muscle, which can throw the body's protein levels out of whack.

Another problem with these quick-loss starvation diets is that the weight is lost more rapidly than what most experts consider to be healthy. Losing weight too fast can disrupt the body's metabolic balance, causing fluid and hormonal shifts that can result in organ damage. Some of the health consequences include long-term problems with the kidneys, short-term heart malfunction, loss of electrolytes, low urinary output, dizziness, headaches, skin problems, and potassium disturbances (which can cause cardiac arrest and death).

Along with these metabolic abnormalities that are brought on by rapid weight loss and starvation, it's important to remember that no food also means a lack of sufficient nutrients. Dieters who severely restrict calories inevitably end up suffering from one or more nutritional deficiencies, whether it's vitamin, mineral, or a combination of the two. Regardless of which diet you choose, it's important to make sure you're still getting your recommended daily allowance of vitamins and minerals (see appendix, p. 197–98, for specific vitamin recommendations). Vitamins A, D, E, and K, for example, are in great supply in animal fats, and totally eliminating these fats from your diet could put you at serious jeopardy of developing a vitamin deficiency that would need to be supplemented with an over-the-counter multivitamin.

Depriving yourself of too much food could make your calorie counts far too short for even the most basic activities. The body has a minimum amount of calorie energy it must consume in order to maintain these simple functions. If the body perceives that you're starving and falling under this mark, it will automatically kick in to energy conservation mode and slow down your metabolism. This slowed metabolism can only make matters worse, so remember that while you'd like to cut down on the calories, reducing them too much can be counterproductive. To understand exactly how many calories you need to consume for weight loss purposes, see "Calorie Requirements" in chapter 6 (page 95).

CHAPTER 4

DON'T BELIEVE THE HYPE

Gimmick Diets Don't Work

The most common question I get from my patients, readers, and viewers pertains to the effectiveness of gimmick diets. There are so many floating around that half the time they have to explain them to me before I can comment. My answer, however, is typically the same—these diets work tremendously well, but only for the authors who are selling millions of copies. Of the thousands of people I've met who have tried one of these diets, medications, or supplements, I can count on one hand how many actually lost weight and kept it off for more than six months. My mother always told me as a child, "There's no shortcut to success." Well, the same can be said about shedding those extra pounds. Losing weight and maintaining that loss require a tremendous amount of motivation, perseverance, and knowledge of your body and its relationship to food.

I hear from chronic dieters all the time how difficult it is not to buy a new diet book or supplement that promises to take off the weight in a matter of weeks. Many of these people have unsuccessfully tried everything from starvation to diet pills, but just like people who spend their last dollar on a lottery ticket, they hold out hope that this new plan will finally be the one that works. The sad truth is that for most people it never does work, and instead of subtracting pounds from their waistline, they add on feelings of inadequacy and depression.

Many of these programs can actually work for a very short period of time if followed strictly. If you're looking to lose ten pounds in a month to look better in a new bikini or the suit you had tailored one size ago, it's difficult to argue against the short-term effectiveness of these plans and medications. However, the key concept to understand here is "short-term." Two of the biggest complaints dieters and doctors lodge against these programs is that they're typically impossible to follow over a long period of time. Then, once you get off one, the weight comes piling back on before you've even had a chance to enjoy looking and feeling better.

Modern society spoils us with conveniences—from automotive transportation to delivery services that bring to your doorstep everything from groceries to movie rentals. This same attitude of "fast and easy" is how people approach weight loss, and it's the biggest mistake you can make with respect to dieting. Those extra twenty pounds didn't appear in three weeks, so it's irrational to hope that they will come off in two (appealing as the idea is). Without a commitment to a lifestyle change that you can sustain, you are doomed to chronic weight fluctuations and disappointment with each new diet or medication that you try.

GIMMICK DIETS

Dr. Atkins's New Diet Revolution: Low-Carb/High-Protein Diets

Dr. Robert Atkins is the creator and promoter of the now famous Atkins diet. There are many other diets that employ a similar strategy of cutting out carbohydrates and loading up on protein and fat, but none have come under as much fire as his diet. Mention the name *Atkins* to many physicians and you immediately see a look of disgust come over their faces. One cardiologist I know was so angered by Atkins's recommendation of high-protein, high-fat foods that he suggested the medical community sue Atkins for the protection of the millions of people who have gone on his program without full knowledge of the possible health consequences.

The centerpiece of the Atkins diet is eliminating carbohydrates from the diet. Carbohydrates include sugars, starch, and cellulose, compounds that you'll find in a variety of foods we regularly eat, such as fruits and vegetables, some dairy products, grains, and beans. Atkins's premise is that most people, especially those who are overweight, are sensitive to carbohydrates, and their body's poor handling of these compounds leads to weight gain. In fact, his theory tries to convince you that these carbohydrates are much more deadly to your waistline than the fats found in fried foods or butter-based lobster sauces.

When you consume carbohydrates, your body breaks them down into the simple sugars such as glucose. Glucose is the body's main source of energy, and it's made available to the cells and organs by the actions of insulin, a hormone manufactured and released into the blood by the pancreas. The insulin floats around the blood and eventually attaches to receptors on the cells. Once the insulin is attached, glucose joins and is offered to the cell to be broken down into energy (adenosine triphosphate, or ATP). Many people, mostly those overweight, suffer from a complicated and not completely understood condition called insulin resistance. For some reason, the cell receptors that bind the insulin aren't able to do so effectively, thereby resisting the insulin and thus preventing it from doing its job of pulling glucose out of the blood and transferring it into the cells. This leads to an excess of circulating glucose and the high blood sugar levels that are often seen in diabetics.

The body doesn't like this excess glucose riding around in the blood, and because the insulin is having a difficult time transferring it into the cells for energy, it eventually gets stored as the enemy—fat. The most common form of fat that this glucose gets converted into is triglycerides, which carry a double dose of trouble—adding on extra pounds and increasing your risk for heart disease. Atkins argues that the body then enters a vicious cycle in which the body responds to the insulin resistance and the inefficient handling of glucose by commanding the pancreas to pump out even more insulin. Not only do you have this excess insulin, but if you continue to consume carbohydrates, even more insulin is produced and the glucose that results from the breakdown of carbohydrates is converted into fat.

So what does Atkins recommend? Restrict your carbs and you can eat as much protein and fat as you want. That means no bread with your cheeseburger, but you can have as many bacon cheeseburgers as you like. Forget about many of your favorite processed foods such as cookies, brownies, pies, ice cream, and nondiet soft drinks—according to the Atkins plan, these foods are loaded with those bad carbohydrates that eventually lead to weight gain. Instead, bring on the lobster smothered in creamy butter sauce, porterhouse steak, and bacon and eggs. These foods are full of fats, but they don't have the carbohydrates—the main culprits, in Atkins's view of fat accumulation.

Though Atkins claims that millions have benefited from his diet, it's well known that his theory of weight gain and dietary recommendations have long cut across the grain of the medical establishment. Scientists will argue energetically about the scientific veracity of his theories about excess insulin and the processing of glucose. However, what has most doctors, dietitians, and health advocates up in arms is the potential health risk dieters place themselves in when following his dietary recommendations. Atkins's theory also relies on a process called ketosis, a state in which the body doesn't get enough of its typical fuel source—glucose—and as a result starts burning fat for fuel. On the surface, that sounds like a great idea. After all, the mission here is to shrink those fat cells—but you should know about the risks of such a counterintuitive approach.

While a body in ketosis will burn the fat and produce ketones—an alternate source of body fuel when glucose is in short supply—it is an unnatural state that the body is neither accustomed to nor easily able to achieve. Ketosis is a process that occurs in more emergent situations, when other body systems are out of whack, and in and of itself can present problems. It can lead to fatigue, nausea, vomiting, and dehydration. Ketones can disrupt the body's important acid-base balance, in some cases increasing the risk for coma and death.

There's also the issue of heart disease, one you'd expect to be of supreme importance to a cardiologist like Atkins. He claims that even though you're allowed to eat as many saturated fats and cholesterol-rich foods as you desire, your total cholesterol levels will drop because the pool of triglycerides will shrink. But not so fast—experts argue that while triglycerides might drop, the bad cholesterol—LDL—will rise, and this alone can increase the risk for heart disease and the formation of atherosclerosis, where plaque builds up along the inner walls of blood vessels. In fact, study after study has shown that one of the highest-risk populations for heart attack is people who are overweight, insulin resistant, and battling high levels of LDL cholesterol.

The Atkins food group distribution stands in contradistinction to that recommended by the USDA (see appendix, page 194). The USDA recommends a diet that consists of 55–65 percent carbohydrate, 20–30 percent fat, and 10–15 percent protein. The Atkins diet completely disrupts this balance, reducing the carbohydrate percentage to practically nothing and increasing fats and proteins to levels that are 75 percent more than what the government recommends for nutritional balance and safety.

The fruits and vegetables that Atkins restricts are staples in our diet and important sources of vitamins, minerals, and other nutrients. Drastically reducing them along with whole grains and dairy products can easily lead to nutritional deficiencies. Atkins does suggest a group of vitamins and supplements to replace these nutrients, but this doesn't provide total protection against possible complications such as dehydration, hypotension (abnormally low blood pressure), and osteoporosis.

Excess protein consumption is another major concern, especially as it might affect the liver and kidney. These two organs are largely responsible for handling the protein, so the concern is that too large of a protein load will overwork them and lead to liver or kidney failure. Some experts have also raised the concern of increased homocysteine levels as a result of the increased animal protein consumption. Homocysteine is an amino acid that has drawn a lot of attention lately, as it's been connected to an increased risk for heart attack and Alzheimer's disease.

Another major criticism about the Atkins diet and many other gimmick diets is that they're almost impossible to stick with for any substantial period of time, which may be the reason why so many people who have tried the diet escape serious injury.

I remember going out with one of my cameramen on a story one afternoon, and as we were riding in the car he looked at me and said, "Hey, Ian, have you noticed anything different?"

I looked him up and down, thinking it was a trick question. "Not really," I replied. A smirk started to spread across his face. "What is it?" I finally asked, realizing he wasn't going to reveal the information unless I specifically asked.

"Wait till we get out of the car," he replied, now a full smile filling his face. When we arrived at the shoot and got out, he opened his coat.

Now typically, he was a moderately overweight man of average height, with a noticeable potbelly. He still had the belly, but it was somewhat smaller, and his pants were actually gapping around his waist.

"How did you do it?" I asked.

"The Atkins diet," he exclaimed. "I've been on it for three weeks and I've already lost sixteen pounds."

"So what have you been eating?" I asked, sizing him up.

"Everything—eggs and bacon, cheeseburgers and fries, steaks—anything I want except for carbs. It's the best diet in the world."

"What about exercise?" I asked, knowing he wasn't exactly the exercising type.

"Not a lick," he replied, taking delight in knowing how much I believed in physical activity and exercise for long-term weight management.

Between my vacation and his vacation and being assigned different shoots, I didn't see him for the next couple of months. When we were finally partnered again, the first thing I did was take a look at his abdomen. Given his previous dramatic weight loss, I expected him to practically have a flat six-pack by now. Needless to say, it was just the opposite. He was not only back to his old size, he looked a little bigger. Before I could say something, he confessed that he was no longer on the diet and had regained the weight plus some. His major reason: The diet was too difficult to follow, and while it was all right to restrict carbs the first few weeks, he found it almost impossible to continue eating that way and eventually returned to his prior eating habits.

My cameraman's short success and ultimate failure on the Atkins diet is an extremely common experience for many who try it. The cornerstone of any good diet or weight control plan must be that it fits a person's individual tastes and abilities and fosters long-term lifestyle changes rather than quickie weight loss strategies.

You may know someone who has lost weight on the Atkins diet, in which case you might be wondering, If there's so much bad associated with it, how do some people actually lose weight on the diet? It really has to do with calories. Almost half of the calories Americans consume daily come from carbohydrates. If you eliminate these calories from your diet, even increasing your fat and protein consumption won't likely add enough calories to replace the deficit incurred by excluding carbs. For example, let's say you typically consume 2,500 calories a day and about 1,250 of those calories come from carbohydrates, while the remaining 1,250 come from fats and proteins. If you eliminate the carbs completely, you're now eating only 1,250 calories a day. The Atkins diet says feel free to increase your protein and fat—but let's say even then you consume only 600 more extra calories with these additions. Your new daily caloric intake now stands at 1,850, still 650 below your typical consumption and enough for you to lose just over a pound every week—and that's without even increasing your energy expenditure through physical activity or exercise. This is why critics prefer to call these low-carbohydrate diets low-calorie diets in disguise. Whether you eliminate carbs from the diet or eat smaller portions of food, the bottom line is you're reducing the caloric intake, and that's what works at the end of the day.

To his credit, Atkins does devote at least a few pages to the benefits of exercise, but the amount of time he gives the subject makes it seem like an afterthought. By the sheer volume of pages he dedicates to explaining his diet and tips on how to remain on it, you are quickly clued in to what he considers most important. Any diet book that talks only about ways of burning the fat through eating habit changes is telling you just half the story. Exercise should be a key component to any diet program that's attempting to not only shed excess pounds, but improve the quality of one's life.

The Zone Diet

Medical researcher Barry Sears and coauthor Bill Lawrence described their diet in a best-seller that topped the charts for weeks and remains a widely-popular diet. Many have been confused by this diet, and I myself had to read it closely to follow their scientific explanations. Even after finally understanding what they were saying, I had serious doubts in my mind. If you were to read the diet's prescription and basis, you might feel the same way.

Like the Atkins diet, one of the Zone's guiding principles is that carbohydrates, not fats, are the major cause of our expanding waistlines over the last few decades. The Zone's overarching theory is that dieters should think of food as a powerful drug rather than a source of pleasure or hunger relief. Sears contends that food should be eaten "in a controlled fashion and in the proper proportions as if it were an intravenous drip." By eating food in precise amounts at specific times, you can alter your hormonal balance, thus sending yourself into a near euphoric state, aptly called the Zone. The Zone is a state in which weight loss is almost automatic; your mind is sharp, yet relaxed; and your muscles work optimally. How do you get to the Zone? Sears conveniently directs you through a dietary road map—but you must follow the instructions carefully to stay there.

Like the Atkins diet, the Zone also disrupts the governmental recommendation for food group distribution. Sears suggests reducing your intake of carbohydrates to 40 percent of your total calories, while the USDA recommends as much as 60 percent. The Zone says protein consumption should equal 30 percent double that of the USDA recommended 15 percent. The USDA recommends a maximum of 30 percent from fats, and the Zone pushes the same maximum, yielding a diet of 40-30-30, carbs-protein-fat.

One of the most controversial components of the Zone is the group of functions it attributes to naturally occurring compounds in the body called "eicosanoids." There is still more to be discovered about the roles these compounds play in the body, but we do know that they play a role in blood clotting and ensuring our immune system works optimally. What hasn't been confirmed is what Sears claims: that they control "every cell, every organ, and every system."

Many scientists have disputed Sears's explanation of "good" and "bad" eicosanoids and have a hard time confirming that they are actually synthesized by this diet. Our current working knowledge suggests that these compounds are synthesized by a series of reactions that start in the membrane, or outer covering, of the cell. Virtually all cells have the ability to form eicosanoids, but the actual amount they synthesize depends largely on the amount of enzymes they contain. These eicosanoids aren't stored in significant amounts like some vitamins; instead, they're manufactured in response to immediate need.

Beyond the difficulties in understanding the science behind the diet, you might meet another major obstacle in figuring out how actually to implement it. To enter the Zone, you must sit down and do several calculations. You must first determine your body's daily protein requirement. Just as with a prescription drug, you're required to divide the daily dose in equal allotments and spread them out over the three meals and two snacks you're supposed to consume each day. Figuring out this daily protein requirement means even more calculations involving your weight, level of physical activity, and percentage of body fat. The book has work sheets to help you with these calculations, but you'll also need a scale and tape measure.

The timing of meals is also extremely important, and you must never allow yourself to go more than five hours without eating. Sears is very clear about what he considers to be diet no-nos. Bad carbs include most grains and breads, ice cream, jelly, all fruit juices, potatoes, peas, corn, carrots, and others. Fiber-rich carbohydrates such as green beans, spinach, blueberries, and apples are acceptable.

Many dietitians and weight loss experts are quick to point out that it's possible to experience a short-term weight loss on the Zone, but this is most likely due to the fact that it's more of a low-calorie diet than anything else. Depending on what you calculate your needs to be, the diet typically consists of 1,000–1,700 calories, which makes it much less than the typical 2,500-calorie American diet.

Sugar Busters

The Sugar Busters diet is the brainchild of three Louisiana doctors and a CEO who collectively blame our excessive sugar consumption for our country's increasing girth. Not unlike the creators of the Atkins diet and the Zone, the authors of this diet contend that the most effective change you can make in your bid to lose weight is to cut the sugar out of your diet. Another similarity—you guessed it—is that you can eat as much as you want of whatever you want as long as it doesn't contain the new age enemy: carbohydrates. The list of sugary foods you must avoid is enormous, and for many dieters it's simply overwhelming. Brown sugar, white flour, white rice, corn syrup, molasses, honey, potatoes, certain pastas, carrots, white bread, pizza crust, cookies, corn, and beets are high on the "don't come near me" list of foods. Why? The explanation again is familiar: The body breaks down these carbohydrates into simple sugars such as glucose, and it's this excess of glucose and hormone production that causes our fat cells to swell.

Sugar Busters does, however, distinguish itself from the Zone in many ways, including the allowance of whole-grain foods. The theory is that the carbohydrate in these foods is acceptable because it's digested more slowly, which keeps the insulin levels relatively lower when compared with levels from other types of carbohydrates. The authors contend that other high-fiber foods—green vegetables, apples, citrus fruits, and dried beans—are all right to eat because they also slow down the production of insulin, which means you can eat larger quantities without gaining weight. Hopefully, you're not a big fruit lover, because if your mouth waters for pineapples, watermelon, or bananas, you're in for a big disappointment on this plan: these high-carb fruits aren't acceptable.

Carnivores will applaud the part of the diet that allows you to eat generous portions of lean meat. You can't have the potatoes with your steak, but you can eat the meat—lean—till your heart and stomach are content. The idea is that the protein in meat stimulates the pancreas to produce glucagon, which, unlike insulin, promotes the breakdown of stored fat.

A major premise of this diet is that by eliminating the "refined sugars"—such as table sugar and the sugar found in processed sweets like candy, cakes, and soda—you will prevent your body from over-secreting insulin, the hormone responsible for converting excess glucose into fat. The problem many critics have with this theory, however, is that there is no scientific proof that a large number of people secrete more insulin than they actually need. In fact, unless you suffer from some type of metabolic disorder or organ dysfunction, the body is actually very efficient at handling all levels of sugar consumption, whether that means making more in the body if we don't consume enough or processing it faster if we consume too much.

Many dietitians will agree that we are consuming too many carbohydrates, but that's not the only story. Along with these carbohydrates, we're consuming high-fat foods, such as fatty meats and rich cream sauces, that lead to weight gain. It's also important not to forget the role that lack of exercise and physical activity have played in expanding our waistlines. The authors make a reference to the importance of participating in moderate workouts for overall fitness and health, but the amount of time they dedicate to this recommendation and their nonenthusiastic tone aren't as convincing as their conviction about the need to restrict sugar consumption.

A team of dietitians has also looked at the calorie count of a typical Sugar Busters diet. Are you ready for this? An average day on the plan provides only 1,200 calories. No wonder this diet might work for some people in the short term; it's nothing more than a low-calorie diet.

Cardiologists are still debating the health claims of the authors. Like Atkins, the Sugar Busters creators claim that by following this diet, not only will the pounds fall away, but cholesterol and triglyceride levels will drop. This remains controversial, but critics also argue that the meats and full-fat dairy products Sugar Busters allows will load up vulnerable blood vessels with artery-clogging saturated fat.

Sugar Busters has been one of the more popular diets over the years, because although it restricts certain foods, it allows you to eat other favorites without stipulating the amount. It doesn't make specific promises about the amount of weight you'll lose, and it doesn't burden you with counting calories and keeping a log of your consumption. Instead it simply says, Don't eat this group of foods, but feel free to eat as much as you want of everything else. Thousands will swear they've lost weight on this diet, but the more important statistic is how many have been able to keep the weight off. Even if you're able to survive on such few calories, what about all the vitamins and minerals you're sure to be missing by eliminating nutrient-rich fruits and vegetables? Losing weight is an important step to improving your health, but doing it by creating a nutritional deficiency is like taking a step forward while at the same time taking a step back.

The Scarsdale Diet

I didn't know much about diets as a boy, always considering them something girls spent too much time worrying about, but I did know a little something about the Scarsdale diet. When the headlines broke that the author of this very popular diet, Dr. Herman Tarnower, cardiologist and founder of the Scarsdale Medical Center in New York, had been killed by his longtime lover and research assistant, the country was in shock. Many women had come to regard the diet and its creator as their personal savior, someone who had made it possible to lose the weight they had been trying to shed for years.

The Complete Scarsdale Medical Diet first hit the shelves in 1979, and even after Tarnower's murder in 1980, the diet remained popular and copies of his book continued to sell briskly. What excited people, mostly women, about the Scarsdale diet was its design to knock off those extra pounds quickly—twenty pounds in fourteen days. This diet really was one of the original crusades for the low-carb, high-protein regimen. Tarnower insisted that dieters consume their major nutrients in specific proportions—carbohydrates (34.5 percent), fat (22.5 percent), and protein (43 percent). This carbohydrate intake is much lower than the USDA's recommendation of 60 percent.

A major premise of the diet is that this specific mix of nutrients was critical in accelerating metabolism, making the body a more efficient burner of fat. Similar to that of the other diets, the aim is to trick the body into entering a state of ketosis, in which fat is burned for fuel and the ketones that are produced suppress the appetite. Tarnower never provided scientific proof for the claims of his diet, instead relying on the testimonials of his many patients who said that they had gone on it and succeeded. It might be just as well that he stayed away from scientifically validating the diet, as it would surely have been contested like many of the other popular diets.

The Scarsdale diet, however, involves more than just cutting back on the carbs and pumping up the protein. It is a low-calorie diet, arguably one of the lowest around, holding the calories to no more than 1,000 a day, half of the average recommended by the USDA. Most nutritionists will tell you that a diet so low in calories is bound to be deficient in certain vitamins and minerals. Without taking some form of supplements, it's almost impossible to consume the necessary amounts from all food groups to supply our bodies with needed energy and nutritional reserves.

Unlike the authors of many of the other programs, Tarnower at least admits that it's not prudent for people to remain on crash diets for long periods of time. Unlike the other diets, in which you're given foods to select from and a great degree of flexibility in how you combine them in your recipes, the Scarsdale diet is built around planned meals that come in several variations, depending on your financial abilities or dietary preferences. You'll spend the first two weeks on a crash diet, then go on a low-carb maintenance program meant not to take more weight off, but to prevent the lost weight from creeping back on. When you're ready to lose more weight, return to the crash diet, severely restricting your calories and eating according to prechosen meal plans.

The Scarsdale diet, while heralded at the time by many of its followers, is fraught with health loopholes that can get dieters into trouble quickly. The diet is designed to alternate between a crash weight loss phase and a maintenance phase—in other words, depending upon a built-in yo-yo component, in which people lose weight, put some of it back on, and then lose more. Earlier, we discussed the dangers of the yo-yo effect and established that weight loss is healthier and more effective when it's carried out gradually.

Excess protein consumption is another concern on this diet. Tarnower recommends that 43 percent of your daily intake comes from protein, while many nutritionists and doctors recommend less than half that amount. Consuming too much protein strains your liver and kidneys—not a good situation if you have a preexisting disease. Protein is important to our bodies, but too much can mean increasing homocysteine, a risk factor for heart disease, or decreasing the amount of calcium available to the body. If your level of calcium remains low for a prolonged period of time, this means an increased risk for osteoporosis—a condition of thinning bones.

One of the major reasons crash diets like the Scarsdale don't work is that the faster you take off weight, the faster you gain it back. You might be able to trick the body by starving it for a short period of time, but sooner or later it becomes wise and makes its own internal adjustments that make it more difficult to lose weight. The Scarsdale diet is another testament to the old adage "There is no shortcut to success."

MEDICATIONS

Wouldn't life be so much easier if a single pill could alleviate all our maladies and discomforts? Imagine this: You step on the scale one morning, and to your horror, you discover that you're carrying an extra twenty pounds. You want desperately to return to a more normal weight, but you've read this book from cover to cover and realize your only chance is to change your relationship with and consumption of food and increase your level of physical activity. Then you hear about a pill just released on the market that will melt the weight away in a month's time.

The truth is that there is no pill that will simply and *safely* burn away those excess pounds.

Fen-phen

Fen-phen is an abbreviation for the combination use of two different medications—fenfluramine and phentermine. Both are FDA-approved drugs; phentermine was given the go-ahead in 1959, while fenfluramine wasn't officially approved until 1973. Dexfenfluramine (Redux) is another drug that has been commonly used in combination with phentermine, appropriately termed dexfen-phen. Like fenfluramine and phentermine, dexfenfluramine is an appetite suppressant used in the management of obesity, and it was officially approved in 1996.

While these drugs were individually approved by the FDA, the combinations that physicians have prescribed in the past—fen-phen or dexfen-phen—have not been approved. But physicians and patients found the drugs to be more effective when combined rather than when taken individually. You might wonder whether physicians were then illegally prescribing these drugs because the FDA hadn't approved of their use in combination. There was nothing illegal about it at all. Physicians reserve the discretionary right to use approved drugs in what's called and "off label" fashion—meaning a drug may not have been approved for a certain condition, but if a physician deems it to be effective and safe, he or she can prescribe it to patients.

Thousands of patients certainly lost a considerable amount of weight with these drug combinations. One of the problems, however, was that no studies were presented to the FDA to demonstrate either the effectiveness or the safety of the drugs taken in combination or over a long period of time. Critics also expressed concern, because most studies involving the drugs' safety were short-term, while the longest large study was a one-thousand-person one-year European study in which half of the patients took dexfenfluramine. Heart disease wasn't noted in the study, but this means almost nothing because doctors were prescribing and patients were taking these medications on a long-term basis.

The proverbial shoe fell on July 8, 1997, when the Mayo Clinic reported twenty-four patients developed heart valve disease after taking fen-phen. Some of these patients eventually required heart valve replacement surgery to correct the condition. This cluster of unusual cases of valve disease in fen-phen users raised a sharp suspicion that there might be an association between fen-phen use and valve disease.

The FDA simultaneously issued a public health advisory that described the Mayo findings. Raising even more concern, the prestigious *New England Journal of Medicine* also reported these findings in the August 28 issue, including an FDA letter to the editor describing additional cases. At the time of the article, the FDA had received over one hundred reports (including the original twenty-four Mayo cases) of heart valve disease associated mainly with fen-phen. There were also reported cases of heart valve disease in patients taking only fenfluramine or dexfenfluramine. Months later, more evidence accumulated about the toxic effects of these drug combinations.

Some of these patients who suffered from valvular heart disease had no symptoms, but many others experienced a combination of symptoms, including shortness of breath, excessive fatigue, chest pain, fainting, and leg swelling. Some physicians heard a new heart murmur when listening to the heart through a stethoscope, while others detected abnormalities on a noninvasive special heart test called an echocardiogram. In fact, in a survey of 291 patients who had received fen-phen or dexfen-phen and didn't exhibit any symptoms of heart disease, 30 percent had abnormal valve findings. Based on all of the reported evidence, the manufacturers agreed to withdraw fenfluramine and dexfenfluramine from the market, and the FDA recommended that patients no longer take the drugs. Phentermine, however, remains on the market, as no cases of heart valve disease that meet the FDA's case definition have yet to be reported.

Water Pills

Diuretics, commonly referred to as water pills, have been taken by thousands of dieters over the years. These prescription drugs are typically given to people who have problems maintaining proper fluid balance and elimination. Patients suffering from congestive heart failure, liver dysfunction, kidney disease, and menstruation-related swelling are often prescribed this class of drugs, and they've proven to be quite effective at assisting the body in eliminating excess fluid. Dieters have latched on to the drugs' success at treating these conditions and self-prescribe it for weight loss. For the most part, dieters can lose large volumes of water weight by taking these diuretics, but the health risks for someone doing it outside of the supervision of a physician are astronomical.

Diuretics can cause permanent damage to your sense of hearing and impairment in your balance system. Excessive water loss can lead to dehydration and all of the events that can follow when your body doesn't have the appropriate amount of circulating blood. The concern, even for medical patients, is that these drugs can cause a depletion of potassium, which can trigger several catastrophic bodily events, including heart attack. Diabetics must be careful when taking these medications, because they can lead to elevated blood sugar levels. Some patients have been taken off diuretics because they can increase the amount of calcium in the body, which can lead to cognitive changes such as agitation and confusion.

Diuretics can be safe drugs, but only when used for a specific medical condition and under the supervision of a health professional who can periodically monitor certain blood chemistries. While these drugs can't be purchased over-the-counter, dieters have been able to access them quite easily. It's silly to put your life at risk by taking a medication that hasn't been approved for weight loss. Cut back on the calories or increase your daily activity and realize even greater health benefits.

Thyroid Pills

Patients who suffer from an underactive thyroid are often prescribed medications that increase the levels of this important hormone. They can help improve several symptoms, including slowed heart rate, low tolerance for cold temperatures, mental sluggishness, and hair loss. The challenge, however, is maintaining the delicate balance between too little and too much thyroid hormone, trying to find a comfortable place in the middle.

Dieters take thyroid hormone for its effect on metabolism and the body's ability to expend energy. Along with all of the important functions of this hormone, it can increase these properties, which can lead to weight loss and a more efficient and easier method of burning energy. In fact, patients who suffer from hyperthyroidism often mention how much weight they've lost without even trying. This sounds like a perfect solution for someone whose metabolism is slowed for some reason or wants to increase their energy burn without increasing their physical activity. The reality, however, is that thyroid pills are far from magic bullets, but instead carry severe side effects such as increased heart rate and heart rhythm disturbances that can be life-threatening. Again, it's critical to never take a medication that hasn't been prescribed specifically to you. It's also important not to use medications that have been prescribed for a specific medical condition for other purposes such as weight loss. The hidden dangers far outweigh the benefits you might expect to receive.

Meridia

Meridia, also called sibutramine hydrochloride monohydrate, is an antiobesity medication that was approved by the FDA in February 2001. Patients typically start with a four-week course of 10 mg per day. If there's inadequate weight loss and the patient doesn't have any medical problems, doctors can advance the dose to 15 mg per day. The 5 mg dose is prescribed for those patients who can't tolerate the higher dose and experience unpleasant side effects. As long as there isn't a reason why the patient shouldn't, doctors might advance the dose to 15 mg per day.

According to the manufacturers, Meridia works by affecting the appetite control centers in the brain. It works through a series of steps to make the brain neurotransmitters norepinephrine, serotonin, and dopamine more readily available. It's unclear exactly how these chemicals affect our feeling of satiety, but patients who have them at increased levels seem to experience a reduction in their appetite and hunger patterns.

While you'll hear some patients swear Meridia has helped them lose the weight they've never been able to lose before, don't get your expectations too high. Meridia isn't a drug for everyone; in fact, it's intended for use in patients who are considered obese (BMI of 30 or greater) or for those with a BMI of 27 or greater who also have diabetes or hypertension.

Even the manufacturers will admit that Meridia isn't a magic pill for weight loss. They strongly encourage patients to make the appropriate lifestyle changes—reducing calorie consumption and getting an appropriate amount of physical activity. The weight loss experts I've spoken with who prescribe Meridia to their patients agree that the drug won't work by itself and that without these additional changes, patients will only face another dieting failure.

One of the biggest reasons doctors are reluctant to prescribe Meridia is its notorious side effects. In several studies, Meridia 5–20 mg once daily was associated with average increases in systolic and diastolic blood pressure of approximately 1–3 mm Hg relative to those who didn't take the drug. There were, however, patients who experienced more substantial increases in blood pressure, which is why anyone prescribed Meridia must have regular blood pressure monitoring by a physician. There was also an increase in the heart rate of four to five beats per minute. Patients should also be aware that the safety and effectiveness of Meridia haven't been determined beyond one year.

The side effects of a particular drug aren't just minor inconveniences that are written in small print at the bottom of the packaging insert. They're real and can be extremely uncomfortable, and patients must weigh this in their decision of whether or not to take the drug. Many patients who have taken Meridia for a period of time have complained about an increase in headaches, dry mouth, constipation, and insomnia. There are other patients, however, who have complained about stomach cramps and severe diarrhea. Once again, patients must decide if they're willing to subject their bodies to these potential alterations in an attempt to lose weight—that is, to achieve what is by no means a guarantee.

Then you must consider all of the drug's contraindications—doctor lingo for those conditions in which the drug should never be taken. Earlier we discussed how disturbing it was to discover that the drug raised both the systolic and the diastolic blood pressures, so obviously those with uncontrolled or poorly controlled high blood pressure shouldn't be prescribed this diet drug. The FDA warns that it also shouldn't be administered to those taking antidepressants that belong to the family of monoamine oxidase inhibitors. Patients who suffer from the eating disorder anorexia nervosa should see a physician and be treated for that condition rather than receive Meridia. If you're taking other centrally acting appetite suppressant drugs, you also shouldn't take the drug. Patients with glaucoma and/or heart disease should avoid the diet drug because of its potential to worsen these conditions.

In evaluating any drug, it's important to realize that the studies and information presented to the FDA are only as good and complete as their architecture and execution. It's almost impossible to discover every side effect or contraindication before the FDA grants its approval. The FDA takes the preponderance of evidence and includes several factors in their decision to approve a drug. Meridia hasn't been on the mass market long enough to have established a detailed history of potential problems, but scientists consider the ingredients of a drug and the way it works to determine if there are still some yet undiscovered conflicts.

The list of "precautions" that should be considered before taking Meridia is quite extensive and includes pulmonary (lung) hypertension, seizures, gallstones, kidney/liver dysfunction, and interference with cognitive and motor performance. There's no overwhelming evidence that Meridia will cause these conditions, only that it has the potential to do so based on its contents and the way it interacts with the body. Physician and patient together should discuss all risks before including Meridia as part of a weight loss regime.

Many physicians insist that they will use Meridia with their patients only when all other mechanisms have failed.

Does Meridia actually work? The manufacturers report that, as happens with many other medications and programs, most of the weight will be lost gradually, during the first six months of therapy. Studies that lasted one year claim that many people who lost weight and remained on Meridia therapy maintained their weight loss. If you take a closer look at the FDA papers on Meridia, however, the story is not promising. In a two-year, double-blind, placebo-controlled trial, the mean weight loss at six months for those taking Meridia was twenty-one pounds, while those not taking Meridia lost only twelve pounds.

Looking at the same people over twelve, eighteen, and twenty-four months, those taking Meridia kept off more of their weight than the others, but in both groups much of the weight was regained. At the end of the study, most patients lost only 5 percent of their initial body weight, half of what experts believe is necessary to reduce the risk of obesity-related complications. When the patients were reexamined a month after the study had completed, those on Meridia had regained double the amount of those who weren't on the drug.

Meridia isn't a cheap drug. Depending on where you purchase it and how strong the dose, expect to pay anywhere from $100 to $200 for a one-month supply. Eating a healthy diet, reducing your caloric intake, and increasing your physical activity is a much less expensive and far safer solution.

WEIGHT LOSS is a lifelong adjustment. This is something you'll hear several times throughout this book, because it should be the guiding principle of any honest and meaningful weight loss program. So if you're on a diet drug for some period of time and your weight has bounced up and down, the inclination is to either quit taking it or simply take it for a longer period of time. That begs an important question—how long should you take Meridia? I'll leave the subject of Meridia with the one line in the FDA approval draft that immediately caught my attention: "The safety and effectiveness of Meridia, as demonstrated in double-blind, placebo-controlled trials, have not been determined beyond 2 years at this time."

CHAPTER 5

EXTREME MEASURES

Surgery As An Option

W hen I was in my third year of medical school at the University of Chicago, I spent two months rotating on the general surgery service. My attending physician was one of only a few bariatric (obesity) surgeons in all of Chicago, specializing in performing surgeries to help those considered morbidly obese. I remember him explaining to his students why he chose to help these people and also why so many of his colleagues frowned upon his practice. The surgical treatment for obesity has been controversial since it first arrived in the early 1950s, and despite its increasing popularity in certain surgical circles, it continues to have its fair share of detractors.

The first surgery I assisted on as a medical student was conducted on a six-hundred-plus-pound woman who had tried practically every diet, supplement, and medication that had been on the market. Despite years of struggling to lose the weight, there she sat in her hospital bed, uncomfortable, crying, and ashamed that she had allowed herself to reach such an unhealthy size. Surgery, in her words, was her last option. All she needed was a little help, something that would allow her to start losing the weight and make it more difficult to put it back on.

My attending physician was always sympathetic toward the many people who came to his office and poured out their souls about years of chronic dieting, temporary successes, and many more disappointments. It's difficult not to imagine the physical and psychological pain these patients endure on a daily basis. Their lives have been dominated by an obsession with food and weight loss, and for many, the psychological wounds can be as debilitating as their physical condition.

My attending physician emphasized, however, that there was one rule that could not be violated. Patients seeking surgical relief had to show they were truly committed to making the lifestyle changes necessary to lose the weight and keep it off. It became important for us to assess not only the patient's physical and psychological problems, but his or her history and efforts at losing the weight through dietary changes and increased physical activity. If patients hadn't demonstrated a sincere effort to lose weight or an ability to handle the challenge of keeping the weight off after surgery, it was explained to them why they weren't a surgical candidate and what they could do to improve their condition to make surgery a reasonable option.

ARE YOU A CANDIDATE FOR SURGERY?

Obesity surgery isn't just for anyone who desires to drop a few dress sizes or has the disposable cash sitting around to pay for it. It's not a cosmetic surgery such as a face lift, where you can walk into a plastic surgeon's office with enough money and pay to have those wrinkles disappear. Weight loss–promoting surgeries are serious interventions that may carry great promise but can also carry tremendous risks. Fortunately, most patients undergoing these procedures don't experience these severe complications, but if you're the unlucky patient who does, the statistics of others' successes become irrelevant to you.

Candidates should also be evaluated by more than just the surgeon. Psychological assessments and counseling can be important in detecting and treating mental afflictions that might be contributing to the weight problem and potentially hindering treatments that could offer a chance at permanent weight loss. Surgery should be reserved for those committed and capable of permanent weight loss. Unlike medications or gimmick diets that can be stopped and started at will, surgery involves internal physical alterations that can also be reversed, but only with considerable health risks and recovery time. This is why surgeons and other members of the health team must be convinced that a candidate is not only physically prepared to handle the rigors of surgery, but mentally ready to take advantage of the weight loss kick start the operation can offer.

Several studies have confirmed the important role surgery can play in those morbidly obese patients who've had such a difficult time shedding unwanted and dangerous extra pounds. Researchers have extensively studied the physical progress of patients who have tried typical weight loss strategies of behavior modification, diet, exercise, and/or medications. It's been made abundantly clear that those considered to be morbidly obese don't lose enough weight just on the traditional weight loss programs to significantly improve their overall quality of life or reduce the associated medical complications and death rate.

How do you know if you're an appropriate candidate? Many bariatric surgeons follow several guidelines, most of which are set in place and agreed upon by the International Federation for the Surgery of Obesity. The first criterion involves weight. Patients must have a present or previously documented BMI of 40 kg/m² or greater, which is approximately one hundred pounds more than your ideal body weight according to the standard height/weight tables. If, however, you don't have a BMI of 40 but measure close to it, you still can be considered a candidate for surgery if the excess weight is causing you to suffer from associated medical or psychological problems such as diabetes, severe sleep apnea, heart disease, and depression. In these cases, it's typically left to the surgeon to decide if, when all things are considered, the benefits of the surgery convincingly outweigh the risks and whether the patient is an appropriate surgical candidate.

In addition to obesity-related medical problems and their severity, other considerations must be made before determining whether surgery is right for you; these include assessing your mental stability, and undergoing a psychological evaluation can be critical in detecting other issues that need to be addressed before surgery becomes an option.

It's also important for doctors to ascertain a substance abuse history—if there is one—and for patients to be honest about their affliction. A history of excessive ingestion of alcohol or drugs—both illicit and prescription—can be an important benchmark for physicians as they assess potential surgical risk. Even if substance abuse has ceased, it's still possible that permanent physical damage has been done that could put a patient at great surgical risk. The request for a full disclosure of a history of alcohol or drug abuse is not used to pass moral judgment, but rather to protect candidates from undergoing a procedure that could be potentially life-threatening.

Patient expectations, so crucial to the success of any weight loss treatment, must be fully explored before obesity surgery is undertaken. There is no magical cure for obesity or shortcuts to shed those excess pounds. Patients must accept the reality that losing weight is going to require a serious commitment and major alterations in lifestyle. Determinations to eat healthier, make behavior modifications, and increase the level of physical activity are critical to success. The need for the patient's determination and commitment to losing weight is discussed many times while investigating the possibility of obesity surgery. Too many potential medical complications are associated with these surgeries to perform them on someone whose commitment is halfhearted. These commitments are tied directly to expectations, as many people falsely believe that surgery is an automatic weight loss method that requires minimal time and effort. A tremendous amount of weight can be lost after the surgery, but that weight will return if the health team's prescription for a healthier way of living is not closely adhered to.

The patient's willingness to comply with all of the pre- and postsurgical requirements set forth by doctors and nutritionists is supremely important. Surgery is a major step, and the demands it places on one's body, mind, and time can be tremendous. A surgeon might want a patient to lose a certain amount of weight before surgery to demonstrate that he or she is truly committed to losing the weight. Weight loss prior to the surgery can also be important in reducing potential surgical complications, and doctors are just as enthusiastic as the patient for a successful operation. There is a critical recovery time from these surgeries, largely because the anatomy has been either reconstructed or drastically altered. During recuperation, patients need to take certain medications, eat a certain diet, administer adequate self-care, and attend follow-up sessions with their doctor, nutritionist, and in some cases, a counselor. If one is not willing to follow this stringent routine, thinking that once the surgery is over the rest will take care of itself, then other options need to be considered.

A reliable support network is an important component for anyone attempting to lose weight, especially those who plan on undergoing surgery. There are times before and after surgery that patients will need spiritual as well as physical support. Many severely obese patients are already physically debilitated and experiencing a significant disruption in their daily functioning secondary to the excess weight and associated medical conditions. The surgery, at least for a time, will likely worsen this decreased functioning as the patient is restricted by the demands of recovery. Having a person or group of people who can be called on to help carry out activities such as doing the laundry, lifting heavy furniture, or performing errands is instrumental. Many patients don't succeed in their efforts to lose weight because they don't have that someone there who can provide that critical assistance.

Surgery is by no stretch of the imagination a walk in the park. It is extremely disruptive to the body's state of natural existence and can place greater demands on patients than what was anticipated prior to the surgery. Some patients can initially experience depressed mood after the surgery, especially as their diet might be changed to liquids only and they remain hospitalized for at least a week to monitor any potential problems in the immediate postsurgical period. Having someone who can hear concerns and understand the difficulties can mean the difference between a successful weight loss program and one that produces only slight improvement.

Despite the rumors that surgery is the only way to achieve permanent weight loss, one must ask oneself some serious questions about previous attempts to lose weight. Chronic dieters who have flipped from one "quick loss" program to another typically have a history of failed weight loss efforts. Whether or not a patient has attempted to lose weight on a plan that incorporates healthy dietary changes, behavior modifications, and increased physical activity will be carefully assessed. If a person has not attempted a more disciplined program that includes lifestyle modifications, then he or she hasn't made a genuine effort to succeed, thus eliminating surgery as an option. Many dieters have tried numerous programs, but their expectations are so unrealistic or out of proportion to their actual efforts that when they fail to see a large weight loss in a few weeks, they deem the program ineffective and search for another. If this profile fits you, then you haven't yet exhausted all potential weight loss options that don't include surgery.

In order to decide if surgery is the best option, one must do some homework. One of the most important components of treatment success is the patient's knowledge of his or her condition and the available therapies that exist. I'm not suggesting that people need to diagnose and treat themselves, but it is certain that a well-informed patient can make better decisions than one who blindly follows the advice that others proffer. First, one must understand how the surgery is performed and why it's supposed to be effective, as well as its benefits and complications. This is basic knowledge that anyone should obtain regardless of what type of surgery is being considered. The only way to make a good decision is to make an informed one, and if one doesn't ask the questions and insist on the answers, one is blindly putting one's health at serious risk. There are several types of obesity surgeries, and individual surgeons use different materials and techniques. Familiarizing oneself with all of these procedures and discussing them with a surgeon with regard to one's medical history and other relevant factors will help determine which type of surgery has the highest possibility of success.

HOW YOUR BODY DIGESTS FOOD

Before one can understand how these surgeries might assist with weight loss efforts, it's critical to have a basic understanding of how the body actually digests food and beverages. It all really starts in your eyes and nose. When you prepare to eat food, whether it's a bag of potato chips or a full meal, your eyes immediately send messages to your brain, which in turn sends messages along the nerves to your mouth and other organs to prepare for food ingestion. Your nose sniffs the wonderful aromas, and this too sends a message to your brain that a tasty meal is on the way and to get ready to digest it. Glands in the mouth quickly ready themselves to secrete hormones and enzymes that, along with your teeth and tongue, will take the first step of breaking down the food into smaller portions that can be transported farther down the digestive tract and eventually digested.

Your tongue pushes the chewed and partially broken-down food to the back of the throat and into the esophagus, the muscular tube that connects the mouth to the stomach. Strong contractions aid the force of gravity in propelling the food down the esophagus and into the stomach. The entire stomach can hold approximately four cups of food or liquid. Children have smaller stomach capacities, which is why they require several meals throughout the day to meet their food requirements.

While the stomach is the first large organ to start to see the meal, a limited amount of digestion actually occurs here. Only proteins are significantly digested by the stomach acid and enzymes that work intensely to break the chemical bonds that hold them together. Within two to four hours after eating, the meal is ready to leave the stomach— partially digested, but still requiring more work before the body can take full advantage of the hidden nutrients. The stomach now releases the food into the first part of the small intestine, the duodenum, by slowly squirting small amounts of food through the opening between the end of the stomach and beginning of the duodenum.

The small intestine constitutes most of the gastrointestinal tract, measuring almost ten feet. You're probably wondering how ten feet of anything can fit into our abdomens, but that's part of the genius of how our amazing bodies have been packaged. The small intestine is coiled into many convenient loops that allow it to be stored efficiently within our bodies. Most of the digestive process occurs in the small intestine, and it's here the important nutrients are absorbed through the intestinal lining and into the bloodstream. Approximately 95 percent of the food energy from protein, carbohydrate, fat, and alcohol is absorbed through the small intestine.

The small intestine is divided into three segments, the duodenum (approximately ten inches), the jejunum (about four feet), and the ileum (around five feet). The small intestine is considered "small" not, obviously, because of its length, but rather because of its narrow diameter, typically measuring an inch across. Its role in human digestion is anything but small. Most of the absorption occurs in the first part— the duodenum—and the first half of the second part—the jejunum. Critical hormones and enzymes mix with the food in these portions of the intestine, leading to the greatest nutrient absorption.

The meal remains in the small intestine for approximately three to ten hours before it begins its final descent through the large colon, which typically measures 3.5 feet long and is separated into five segments (cecum, ascending colon, transverse colon, descending colon, and sigmoid colon). The small intestine has typically done such a good job of digesting the meal that little remains for the large intestine. There are often remnant plant fibers—typically difficult to digest— that are attacked by the important bacteria that live in the lower part of our guts. What's not digested by the final efforts of the large intestine remains for another twenty-four to seventy-two hours before being eliminated. Surgeons use the principles of the gastrointestinal tract's anatomy and function to assist them in devising techniques that will help reduce the amount of food consumed and what's eventually digested.

BARIATRIC SURGERY TECHNIQUES

The first surgery for obesity was performed in 1952, and there have been many developments since that have made these surgeries safer and more effective. There have been essentially two prototype surgeries that have been accepted by the National Institutes of Health. The first is called "vertical banded gastroplasty," or what is commonly referred to as stomach stapling. In these procedures, the surgeons operate on only one organ, the stomach. The second category of operations is known as the Roux-en-Y gastric bypass. This procedure involves surgery on the intestine as well as the stomach. Both types of procedures, the methodology behind them, and their intended results are described in the next two sections.

Gastric Stapling/Banding

Gastric stapling/banding divides the stomach into a tiny upper pouch and a large lower pouch. While these pouches are created, a dime-size opening between the two is preserved so that food can pass from the upper to the lower pouch. Depending on the surgeon's preference, the stomach is divided by a series of staples, then a band is sewn into the stomach to reinforce the constriction of the outlet between the pouches that helps prevent it from stretching open. Surgeons might choose to use different materials to form the band, but the physical separation remains the important surgical result.

This partitioning of the stomach virtually reduces its effective size. The idea behind it is simple—when you eat, the tiny upper pouch fills faster than normal. This fast distension produces a feeling of fullness and satiety, sending a message to the brain that the hunger has been appropriately satisfied. In the earlier versions of this surgery, patients found that after a period of time, they began requiring more food to reach that feeling of fullness. Most likely, the opening between the two pouches had stretched to the point that the upper and lower parts had become one. This, of course, defeated the intention of the surgery. As a result, doctors have since tried all types of materials and techniques to prevent the opening from stretching. Newer technical modifications and better patient education have helped alleviate most of these problems, but many surgeons are still reluctant to perform this procedure.

The medical literature about the success of this procedure reveals that the results can vary widely. Dr. Edward Mason, who developed the procedure at the University of Iowa, reports amazing results—five years after the procedure, 50 percent of his patients maintained a 50 percent excess weight loss and 40 percent kept this weight off ten years after the procedure. A Swedish study reported more modest results, showing that 80 percent of the patients experienced a 25 percent loss of their excess weight five years after surgery.

Others report that while 70 percent of patients experience at least some weight loss, many fail to keep off the extra pounds. While they adapt to eating smaller amounts of food, they begin simply to eat more often throughout the course of the day, effectively consuming the same amount of calories, just spread out over more meals.

Roux-en-Y Gastric Bypass

This surgery is typically more extensive than the gastric stapling or banding procedures and remains popular with many surgeons because of its relatively lower rate of complications compared to other obesity surgeries. It effectively combines two older surgical procedures, gastric stapling and intestinal bypass (an operation where the surgeon alters the anatomy to reduce how much of the intestines the food actually travels through). The surgeon operates on two parts of the body, the stomach and then the intestines. Unlike gastric stapling, where the stomach remains intact but is divided into an upper and lower pouch, bypass surgery actually cuts the stomach into two separate parts, one of which is a tiny pouch that can hold only two to four tablespoons (three ounces) at a time.

The surgeon then cuts the jejunum (second part of the intestines) and reattaches it directly to the small pouch. This means when you ingest food, it goes to this newly created and much smaller stomach, bypassing most of the stomach (which is no longer connected) and moving directly into the jejunum and the rest of the intestines. This surgery accomplishes two important goals. First, the amount of food that you can eat before feeling full is dramatically diminished compared to the normal servings you can tolerate when the stomach is intact. Second, because the food you eat bypasses most of the stomach and the first part of the intestines (duodenum), your body has less time and area to actually absorb the calories of the meal.

BENEFITS OF SURGERY

The potential benefits from obesity surgery are all determined by the patient's ability to develop and maintain the necessary lifestyle adjustments to lose the weight and keep it off. In fact, immediately after surgery, most patients begin to lose weight rapidly. If no complications develop and the patient continues to eat a healthy diet mixed with increased physical activity, there's no reason why this weight loss shouldn't continue for eighteen to twenty-four months after surgery, or in some cases even longer.

Surgery success stories are splattered across the medical literature, highlighting some of the improvements these patients have experienced after surgery. The massive weight loss that can follow surgery resolves most long-term obesity-related hormonal, metabolic, and cardiovascular problems. In a study appearing in the *Journal of Gastrointestinal Surgery*, MacDonald et al. reported that more than 73 percent of patients with type II diabetes no longer required insulin or the oral diabetes medications after surgery. The study went on to say that those who didn't have the surgery had a death rate three times greater than that of the surgical patients. For many diabetic patients, surgery-induced weight loss can be adequate enough to return the blood sugar levels to normal. Obstructive sleep apnea, the debilitating condition of patients waking through the night because of periods of stopped breathing, has long been associated with obesity. Researchers have reported that many of those patients who experienced significant weight loss following the surgery improved; in fact, one study claimed that 90 percent of the participants were cured.

Other medical conditions that have improved after significant weight loss include high blood pressure, high cholesterol, amenorrhea (absent menstruation), sex hormone production, infertility, urinary stress incontinence, and esophagitis (inflammation, irritation, and pain in the esophagus). Beyond these medical problems, obesity predisposes some people to simple functional problems, activities that the rest of us take for granted. When patients lose much of this excess weight and grow accustomed to their new bodies, they find improvements in mobility, being able to tie their shoes, sitting more comfortably, being able to flex forward to pick up objects, caring completely for themselves, maintaining adequate hygiene, fitting into public seating, and buying clothing off the rack. It's been encouraging that many obese patients who were not working are able to rejoin the workforce and again feel productive. For many who have failed in other weight loss programs, surgery could be just the jump start needed to get on the road to a healthy and improved life.

SIDE EFFECTS OF OBESITY SURGERY

All surgeries carry the potential for side effects. The surgical team, including the surgeon, anesthesiologist, and nursing staff, does everything to reduce these complications, but even in the most experienced surgical hands and medical care, problems arise. This is one reason why deciding to have surgery is a major step: even though the aim is to improve one or more medical conditions, the surgery itself can trigger other medical problems. This makes presurgical screening all the more important, and it is essential that doctors exercise careful judgment before operating.

Each type of surgery carries the risk of specific complications, and there are side effects that are shared by both. Patients who undergo the restrictive gastric operations—stapling or banding—find themselves at risk for second operations because the staple line has either broken down or the stomach outlet has been so stretched. Once the opening has been increased, the two pouches are reunified, and the stomach becomes one, defeating the whole intention of the surgery (which is to reduce the amount of food the stomach holds and thereby reduce how much is consumed).

It's important for those who have undergone the stapling or banding surgeries to realize that their stomach capacity has been reduced dramatically. Those who return to eating normal or large-volume meals will find themselves throwing up the food they are unable to hold down. The problem is easily rectified by limiting the volume of food consumed in one sitting and reducing the size of the bites that are taken.

Many patients who undergo the Roux-en-Y gastric bypass quickly learn that it's not a great idea to eat food high in refined sugar (table sugar) and fats. These types of foods enter the small intestine very quickly—dumping—and in some patients this can cause nausea, weakness, sweating, and faintness. Because the amount of intestine that gets a chance to absorb food nutrients is reduced by this surgery, it can take some time for patients to adjust their eating habits and for their bodies to digest the food effectively. While these adjustments are being made, patients might experience diarrhea or increased transit time of food through the gastrointestinal tract.

Beyond their specific concerns, both surgeries share a list of potential complications that must be understood before making the decision to head off to the operating room. One of the major concerns that most doctors and patients have is the need to do a second surgery. Of patients who have weight loss operations, 10 to 20 percent require follow-up operations to correct complications. Abdominal hernias, where an internal structure protrudes through the abdominal wall, are the most common complications requiring surgery.

Gallstones are a major concern, because more than one-third of obese patients who have gastric surgery develop them. These hardened collections of cholesterol and other matter form in the gallbladder like tiny marbles and often need to be surgically removed because of the excruciating pain they can cause or the potential complication of gallbladder rupture. The reason so many patients develop gallstones after surgery has to do with rapid or substantial weight loss. In fact, the risk for developing gallstones is so high for these patients, doctors might remove the gallbladder at the time of the obesity surgery as a means of prevention. If the gallbladder isn't removed, some doctors will prescribe supplemental bile salts for the first six months following surgery, in hopes of reducing the risk.

Significant weight loss is extremely important, but it's important to minimize the nutritional costs. Nearly 30 percent of patients who undergo weight loss surgery develop nutritional deficiencies such as iron-deficient anemia, osteoporosis, and metabolic bone disease. The amount of food that many of these patients consume is drastically reduced after surgery, and the absorption of food nutrients is particularly decreased, especially in patients who have undergone the Roux-en-Y procedure. This is why it's important to eat healthy, nutrient-rich foods full of vitamins and minerals. For many of these patients, nutritional supplements could be beneficial, helping to fill in the gaps of a deficient diet.

One of the biggest things to guard against with all of these obesity surgeries is a false sense of security, believing that the operation will cure all woes and effectively eliminate the need for significant lifestyle changes. Nothing could be further from the truth, and it's this attitude that causes many people who have undergone surgery to regain the weight even after an initial loss. The surgery should not be confused with a license to continue eating unhealthy, fat-rich foods or decline participation in regular physical activity and exercise. It should be viewed as one would the jumper cables of a car—just enough to get the engine to turn over; after that, the rest of the parts must do their share to make sure the car keeps running.

LIPOSUCTION ISN'T A WEIGHT LOSS SURGERY

One of the most common questions I hear from patients and colleagues is whether liposuction surgery will help them lose their unwanted pounds. The answer is a thundering *No!* Liposuction is a procedure in which a plastic surgeon or dermatologist takes a thin, prolonged metal probe and inserts it under the skin to remove fatty tissue in specific areas of the body. It's a completely elective cosmetic surgery, one intended to improve physical appearance. It has no implications for improving your health, and despite widely held misconceptions, it's not an effective method of improving the numbers that register on your bathroom scale.

Most doctors who perform liposuction will readily tell their patients that its purpose is strictly to sculpt the contours of the body and remove pockets of fat that refuse to disappear even with proper exercise and diet. Patients often opt to have fat removed from their abdomens, hips, inner thighs, or arms, but the amount that's removed is relatively minimal, just enough to flatten those areas that were once dimpled by the excessive fat underneath the skin. In fact, many of the complications that have occurred in liposuction patients have been blamed on overly aggressive doctors who actually removed too much fat. Excessive fat removal, just as in extreme weight loss, can be dangerous to patients because it disrupts the natural fluid balance in the body and can lead to severe metabolic disturbances.

The ideal candidate for liposuction is someone who is at or near his or her normal weight, exercises regularly, and eats a healthy diet. This person is not interested primarily in losing weight and doesn't suffer from medical problems such as diabetes or heart disease. Obese or moderately overweight people are not good candidates for liposuction because the amount of fat that is ultimately removed would not be enough to make a noticeable difference. These patients often suffer from other obesity-related illnesses that would best be treated through true obesity surgery or a combination of lifestyle changes. Liposuction should be viewed simply as an artistic procedure where what is already in good shape is made to look a little better.

PART THREE

GET THE SKINNY ON YOUR BODY

CHAPTER 6

THE TRUTH ABOUT ENERGY AND METABOLISM

An important part of being able to visualize your weight control and exercise program is having a basic understanding of exactly what it means when you read or hear the words *energy* and *calorie.* These words and concepts are tossed about freely in the world of dieting but are seldom ever explained in a way that makes sense to the layperson. Can you lose weight without understanding the true definitions of energy and calorie? Of course. But in that case, your actions would simply be robotic. You'd be following a set of instructions that others have prepared without understanding the reasons or consequences of your actions, leaving you at the mercy of a particular regimen rather than empowering you, through knowledge, to take control of your overall diet.

Knowing what you're doing to your body when you choose a high-calorie meal versus one low in calories is all part of boosting your mental advantage. Understanding the physical consequences of biting into that ice cream–covered apple pie can only serve as another deterrent to choosing foods that deliver enormous calorie loads. Knowledge of the relationships among calories, energy, and weight gain will automatically trigger alarms in your head as you consider the pie option on the dessert menu. I like to believe that those with proficient knowledge develop something called the "dieting inner voice" (DIV), a second conscience that's preoccupied with the foods they consume, the activities they participate in, and what effects both have on the waistline, overall health, and quality of life.

DIV works around the clock, constantly battling those other voices of gluttony and uninhibited pleasure. It springs into action most effectively when we have several options to choose from, and at least one that is low in calories and rich in vitamins and minerals—we'll call this the DIV option. Most restaurant menus will have at least one DIV option; for example, you'll commonly be able to order a plate of seasonal fruit, even if it's not listed on the menu. The low-calorie DIV option is effective at not only satisfying that sweet craving most of us have after a meal, but ensuring that we don't ruin a calorie-balanced meal with a dessert that will send our calorie count skyrocketing.

This word—*calorie*—that we like to use so carelessly has a scientific definition not too difficult to understand. Scientists define it as the amount of heat energy needed to increase the temperature of 1 kilogram of water (slightly more than a quart) by 1 degree Celsius. So imagine that you have a pot filled with just over a quart of water. You'd first take the temperature of the water, then record it. Next, you'd turn on the stove and heat the water until that temperature is 1 degree Celsius higher. The amount of heat that you used to increase the temperature is a unit of energy defined as one calorie.

Before we go any further in discussing energy and the way our bodies take in this energy in the form of calories, it is important to remember the basic equations of weight loss. In order to maintain your weight, the energy that goes into your body must be equal to the energy that your body burns. If you want to lose weight, the energy in must be less than the energy out. It then follows that gaining weight means the energy in is greater than the energy out.

energy in = energy out (maintain weight)

energy in < energy out (weight loss)

energy in > energy out (weight gain)

The chemical bonds of carbohydrates, fats, and proteins trap energy that is eventually released inside the body during a series of chemical reactions. The energy is made available to the trillions of cells in our body to carry out the many functions that allow us to live. This energy value of food is expressed in terms of calories, which is why nutritionists and diet experts are always cautioning us to watch the amount of calories that we consume. This calorie system is also convenient for those trying to keep track of what they eat, because the United States Department of Agriculture has already calculated the calorie content for almost all foods. If you look at the back of food labels, you'll usually find the caloric content in one typical serving. (Pay careful attention to how many servings are contained in one package, as many suggested serving sizes are suspiciously diminutive.) Look at the number of calories in a cup of whole milk—160 calories. Compare this to a cup of skim milk—90 calories. If someone who consumed a quart of whole milk each day switched to skim milk, the amount of calories ingested each year would be reduced by an amount equal to approximately 11.4 kilograms, or 25 pounds, of body fat.

Scientists have also made it easy to compare the calories of the three major nutrients, which helps us understand why, gram for gram, fats are your worst enemy. A gram of fat contains a net 9 calories. An equal amount of carbohydrate or protein contains less than half of that value, 4 calories. Regardless of how these gimmick diets try to persuade you that carbohydrates (sugars) are the enemies, the bottom line is that a calorie is a calorie is a calorie. For the same volume of food, a food rich in fat can pack twice the amount of calories. The numbers prove that a small quantity of one food can have the same energy as a much larger volume of another food, or even more. As an example, exercise scientists Frank Katch and William D. McArdle looked at how much you'd have to eat of five popular food groups if you were to consume 100 calories. It would take twenty stalks of celery, four cups of cabbage, or twenty asparagus spears to equal just one tablespoon of mayonnaise or ⅘ tablespoon of salad oil.

BALANCING YOUR ENERGY

Energy is essential to our existence as human beings. Food and beverages are our main sources of energy, similar to the fuel we use in cars. Our body breaks down food through a series of complicated chemical reactions, and the energy that's released is what ultimately gets used for us to live. When we eat more food energy than what our body needs or is capable of using, then that energy gets stored as fat. The key, however, is understanding that the source of the calories doesn't matter. Whether you've consumed a calorie load from vegetables or candy bars, if you don't burn off the energy, your body needs to do something with the extra energy. What it does is store those surplus calories in our adipose tissue. Translation: We become fatter.

CHANGE IN FAT STORES = ENERGY IN – ENERGY OUT

We've already discussed the "energy in" part of this equation, but the more complicated issue is the "energy out" portion, which is appropriately called "energy expenditure." Each day we burn a certain amount of energy that's determined by our resting metabolic rate, thermogenic effect of food, and physical activity.

energy expenditure = resting metabolic rate
+ thermogenic effect of food + physical activity

It's easy to see that you can readily manipulate how much energy you expend by making changes on the other side of the equation. Scientists have actually calculated how most of our energy is consumed and thus have delivered some challenging news to those who prefer to sit on the couch. Between 15 and 30 percent of your calories are burned off through physical activity such as exercising in a gym, climbing the steps in your home, or gardening. The resting metabolic rate is responsible for the largest share of your daily energy expenditure, anywhere from 60 to 70 percent. The smallest component of daily energy burn occurs from the body's actual digesting, absorbing, and processing of food. This dietary-induced thermogenesis is typically responsible for about 10 percent of the day's energy expenditure.

The resting metabolic rate includes three different types of metabolism: basal, arousal, and sleeping.

resting metabolic rate = basal metabolism + arousal
metabolism + sleeping metabolism

The basal metabolism requires the largest amount of energy because it includes all of the involuntary activities that are necessary to sustain life. Digestion and voluntary activities aren't part of basal metabolism, but it does include circulation of blood and lymph, respiration, maintenance of body temperature, hormone secretion, nerve activity, and synthesis of new tissue such as skin or the daily turnover of the lining of our gastrointestinal tract.

Even while we're sleeping our body continues to breathe, circulate blood, undergo muscle contractions, and perform other functions. However, when we're asleep the body enters a dormant state and strives to conserve energy; these functions occur at a much slower rate and thus require less energy than when we're awake. When we get up from resting, this arousal is considered to be an added energy expense. It constitutes the smallest part of our metabolism, but it requires energy nonetheless and contributes to our daily energy expenditure.

As mentioned in previous chapters, there's little we can do, if anything at all, to increase our resting and basal metabolism. We typically operate within a specific range, and much of this is determined by the genes we're born with. We also have little control over the energy that's burned owing to our eating of certain foods. This too remains within a tight range, but some studies interestingly show that some nutrients require more energy to digest than others. The body must expend a larger than normal amount of energy to digest protein, which is why some have argued for a high-protein diet for those trying to lose weight. The argument that a protein-rich meal makes fewer calories available to the body and thus decreases the ultimate calorie load does have scientific validity. This interesting phenomenon, however, is exploited by many weight loss diets and overhyped supplements that claim eating certain foods can elevate your dietary-induced thermogenesis and ultimately your basal metabolic rate. The truth is that any meal will temporarily boost your metabolism, but this boost peaks within the first hour after the meal and decreases back to baseline soon thereafter. The noted metabolic boost differences among the food types isn't great enough for you to take notice, and certainly not dramatic enough for many of these diet promoters to make such grandiose claims. Another point not to forget, especially as it relates to high-protein diets, is that high levels of protein can eventually lead to liver and kidney disorders.

The part of the energy equation that we have the most control over involves our level of physical activity. Approximately eight hours a day are spent in resting activities as defined by the resting metabolic rate, but the majority of time is devoted to an assortment of physical activities, whether it's walking to the store or playing a game of tennis. Depending on the type, duration, and intensity of the activity, we can dramatically increase the "energy out" side of the equation, which ultimately favors weight loss.

Fortunately, you don't have to calculate the amount of energy expended during your daily activities, as this has already been calculated by researchers who have gone to great lengths to perform the various measurements. In "Caloric Expenditure During Various Activities" (see appendix, page 226), you can discover how much energy is burned while performing everyday activities such as brushing your teeth, walking the dog, or driving the car. The important point for many who dislike going to gyms or participating in sports is that traditional exercise, while often the most efficient way to burn calories, isn't the only way.

Let's look at some sample activities and compare their energy expenditures. If a 150-pound person wanted to burn 250 calories in physical activity, he or she could choose from a variety of activities:

Gardening that involves digging: 30 minutes
Shopping: 60 minutes
Car washing: 52 minutes
Ballroom dancing: 36 minutes
Roller-skating: 31 minutes
Racquetball: 21 minutes
Fast ax chopping: 12.5 minutes

These, of course, are only rough estimates, but they're important guidelines nonetheless to help us monitor our energy expenditure. Several factors will adjust these predicted energy values. If you're performing a weight-bearing exercise such as grocery shopping or ballroom dancing, in which you must transport your body mass, the heavier you are, the greater the energy cost of a particular exercise. A 150-pound person burns 250 calories when roller-skating for thirty-one minutes, but a 203-pound person will burn 324 calories in the same amount of time.

Gender also plays a role in the amount of energy that's expended during a particular activity, and not because of outdated beliefs that women are weaker or don't work as hard. The answer resides in the body composition difference between the sexes. Men tend to be leaner, as muscle constitutes a higher percentage of their body composition. The male musculature is also larger, and studies have repeatedly shown that the larger your muscles, the greater the energy requirement to perform activities. This is why I recommend that in addition to increasing your level of aerobic exercise when choosing a physical activity plan, you add some type of strength training that will not only increase your tone, but improve muscle strength. Someone with larger muscles who plays a tennis match with the same vigor as a weaker opponent will inevitably consume more energy throughout the match.

CALORIE REQUIREMENTS

All living things have some requirement for energy. Our greatest source of energy comes in the form of food and beverages. Regardless of how small we are or how little our energy demands may be, there is a minimum amount of calories that we need to stay alive, even if our lives consist only of sitting in front of the TV and breathing. Calorie requirements, of course, can vary dramatically among individuals just as much as our daily activities. Someone who is a construction worker or logger and therefore spends a large portion of time lifting and transporting heavy weights will require more calories to perform such tasks than someone who spends most of the day sitting at a desk in front of a computer screen. The same comparison can be made for a person who walks two miles each evening after work versus another person who rents a movie as the night's only activity.

The national recommendations for energy intake are based on average people. For example, a woman who's approximately 20 years old, stands 5 feet 5 inches, weighs about 128 pounds, has average body fatness, and engages in light activity typically requires 2,200 calories per day. The average male for comparison is 20 years old, stands 5 feet 10 inches tall, weighs 160 pounds, has average body fatness, and is lightly active. He typically requires 2,900 calories per day. These, however, are only averages, which means individual differences can ultimately affect typical energy needs. Taller people need proportionately more energy than their shorter counterparts because their large bodies and thus greater surface area mean more energy can escape as heat. Older people typically need less energy than younger people, because their metabolism is slower and they have less muscle mass.

There is, however, a way for you to figure out what your energy needs are without getting bogged down with too many complicated formulas. First, change your weight from pounds to kilograms (1 lb. = 2.2 kg, so 160 lb. = approx. 73 kg). Next, multiply this number by the BMR (basal metabolic rate) factor of 1 calorie per kilogram per hour—which defines the energy requirement for simple metabolism (73 kg x 1 cal. per kg per hr. = 73 cal. per hour). Then, multiply the calories used in 1 hour by the number of hours in a day (73 cal. per hr. x 24 hr. = 1,752 cal. per day). So, a 160-pound man typically requires 1,752 calories per day just to cover the energy cost of metabolism.

Now you must take into account your daily physical activity. This is recorded as estimates or approximations of energy expenditure based on the amount of muscular work a person typically performs in a day. You should find which description fits your activity pattern and select those values:

SEDENTARY LIFESTYLE: Men, 25–40%; women, 25–35%
You sit down most of the day and drive or ride whenever possible.
LIGHT ACTIVITY: Men, 50–70%; women, 40–60%
You move around some of the time, as a teacher might during working hours.
MODERATE ACTIVITY: Men, 65–80%; women, 50–70%
You engage in some intentional exercise, such as an hour of jogging four or five times a week, or your occupation calls for some physical work.
HEAVY ACTIVITY: Men, 90–120%; women, 80–100%
Your job requires much physical labor, such as a roofer or a carpenter.

EXCEPTIONAL ACTIVITY: Men, 130–145%; women, 110–130%

The exceptional category is reserved for those few who spend many hours a day in intense physical training, such as professional or college athletes during their seasons.

When picking the activity level that best suits you, remember that it's based not on how busy you are during the day, but on how much muscular work you perform, whether digging in your garden, lifting boxes, or climbing several flights of stairs throughout the day.

Once you've picked your activity level, you are ready to calculate your daily energy expenditure by using both the upper and lower ends of the range of percentages given for your gender and activity level. Suppose our 160-pound man participates in moderate activity. We can calculate the energy he expends in his activities by multiplying his BMR by the endpoints of the range—in our example, 65 and 80 percent.

> 1,752 calories per day x .65 = 1,139 calories per day
> 1,752 calories per day x .80 = 1,402 calories per day

This means our man needs between 1,139 and 1,402 calories per day just to fuel his physical activities. Now if you total his metabolic requirements that we calculated earlier with his physical activity requirements, you can calculate the daily energy expenditure.

> 1,752 calories per day + 1,139 calories per day = 2,891 calories per day
> 1,752 calories per day + 1,402 calories per day = 3,154 calories per day

This range of daily energy expenditure shows us just how many calories our man needs to support his day's activities. It's also critical in our being able to figure out the energy equations mentioned earlier that determine whether or not he will maintain the same weight, lose some, or gain. If he eats between 2,900 and 3,200 calories per day, everything else being equal, his weight will remain largely unchanged. The key is that in order for him to lose weight, he must consume less energy than what he actually expends.

ENERGY FROM CARBOHYDRATES

Carbohydrates are typically the most abundant of the three major nutrients in our diets. They come almost exclusively from plants, except in the case of milk, which is the only animal-derived food that contains significant amounts of carbs. If you remember your biology from high school, you might recall that plants synthesize carbohydrates through a process called photosynthesis. The chlorophyll—green pigment of plants—captures the energy from the sunlight. This energy is used to combine the water that gets absorbed through the plants' roots with the carbon dioxide that gets absorbed by the leaves from the environment. The water—H_2O—donates the hydrogen and oxygen, while the carbon dioxide gas—CO_2—donates carbon and oxygen. These atoms combine to form the most common of sugars—glucose.

While we eat plants such as fruits and vegetables for their great supply of glucose energy, we are only getting second dibs. Plants themselves use some of the glucose they make to supply the energy for the work of all of their cells. Luckily for us, however, plants don't use all of the glucose they manufacture, and what remains is available to us once we consume the plant or its fruit.

A carbohydrate, however, contains more than just glucose. It includes two major categories, the three monosaccharides—or single sugars—and the three disaccharides—double sugars. Glucose, fructose, and galactose constitute the monosaccharides, with fructose occurring mostly in fruits. The disaccharides are also important in our nutrition, and all three contain glucose as at least one of their sugar components. They're commonly referred to as lactose, maltose, and sucrose—what is most familiar as table sugar.

The purpose of explaining these different sugars is not to confuse you with their strange names, but to help explain that all sugars aren't created equally. The energy of fruits and many vegetables comes from sugar in the form of fructose, which the body breaks down into glucose. This, however, doesn't mean that eating sweet-tasting fruit is the same as eating those concentrated sweets that many are addicted to, like candy and soda. Processed sugary foods provide the body with sugar in the form of glucose, which the body does not need to break down and which therefore enters the bloodstream almost immediately. Both kinds of sugar provide a large quantity of glucose. The major difference is in what else they deliver. Refined sugars found in sweets are delivered in a concentrated form and provide very little if anything in the way of nutrients. Fruits, on the other hand, deliver fructose diluted in large volumes of water, packaged with minerals and vitamins that are important to our overall health and nutrition; fructose enters the bloodstream more slowly because the body needs to break it down before it can be utilized.

The body gets most of its energy from the three major nutrients—glucose, protein, and fats—but glucose remains the preferred body fuel for all cells. In fact, the nerves running through our bodies and the brain almost exclusively use glucose as their fuel source. When we consume more glucose than our day's energy expenditure requires, the hormone insulin signals the body's tissues to take up the excess glucose. The muscle and liver cells are happy to see this extra supply of glucose because they can store it until the body once again needs another surge of energy. The storage form of this surplus glucose is called glycogen, and once energy demands are placed on the body, the glycogen stores are immediately broken back down into glucose and fuel becomes available to the body.

Another, less desirable result of excess glucose is its conversion into fat. Once the body's energy needs are met, and the glycogen stores are at capacity, the liver takes a third and dreaded pathway of handling the incoming carbohydrate. It breaks down the extra glucose into smaller fragments, then reassembles these fragments into a more permanent form of energy storage—fat. This same process isn't exclusive to excess carbohydrate—excess protein and fat are ultimately broken down and stored in the body's abundant adipose tissue. Excess energy takes anywhere from twenty-four to seventy-two hours to be stored as fat.

ENERGY FROM FAT

Typically, when we read or hear the word *fat* we automatically think of bad things such as obesity, heart disease, and physical discomfort. The truth, however, is that fat is an important part of our existence, helping to form the outer coat of each cell in our body. Fat is also the body's chief form of storage for the excess energy from food when we eat in excess of our energy need. This energy store can serve a critical role when we find ourselves in food deprivation or participating in intense physical activity that makes heavy demands on our muscles. When the demand for energy is high and the supply is low, the body goes through a series of reactions that breaks down the components of fats and releases the much needed energy.

The high volume of energy that fats provide can be both a blessing and, in some instances, a curse. Remember, a single gram of fat provides 9 calories, while a gram of carbohydrate or protein provides only 4 calories. If, for example, you find yourself on an extended outdoor adventure and your food intake will be decreased because of the conditions, fatty foods are important because of the amount of energy they pack. How can people go on a fast, lose weight, yet continue to function (albeit impaired at times)? It all has to do with the body releasing energy from the fat cells. If, however, your diet consists largely of high-fat foods—which, unfortunately, most Americans' diets do— and the energy requirements of your daily physical activities are less than what you consume, here comes the weight gain.

Many of these low-carb, high-fat diets tell consumers that if they're willing to eliminate the carbs from their diets, they can eat as much as they want of other foods, including those rich in fats. Such diets are based on the premise that excess glucose, as mentioned previously in this chapter, gets stored as fat. The carbohydrate must first be broken down into smaller fragments, then these fragments are reassembled into fats. This reassembly actually requires energy, which makes fat storage from glucose an inefficient process. That, however, isn't true for fats. Fats you consume in the diet must also be broken down into smaller fragments before being stored, but this process is more energy-efficient and requires fewer steps—both conditions that the body finds favorable. So when the body sees the same number of calories from excess dietary fat or carbohydrate, the body is more inclined to store more calories from fat than from the carbohydrate. These scientifically validated concepts completely contradict the claims many "diet gurus" make regarding their position that it's better to get your calories from fat than it is from carbohydrate. The available science, which is quite extensive, just doesn't substantiate these claims.

An integral part of any weight management program should include an understanding of how the body uses abundant fat stores as a source of energy.

METABOLISM EXPLAINED

You've heard of the expression "There's no such thing as a free lunch." Well, here's a new one: "There's no such thing as a free breath." Everything you do, whether it's picking up the remote control to turn the channel or chewing a piece of gum, requires your body to expend a certain amount of energy. This energy doesn't just suddenly appear; instead, it comes from a series of complicated chemical processes that require the transformation of food or stored energy. These chemical processes constitute our metabolism.

> **METABOLISM:** all the physical and chemical processes by which living organized substance is produced and maintained, and also the transformation by which energy is made available for the uses of the organism.

Metabolism is another one of those fancy words we often hear when people are discussing diets. It's an overused word that's not well understood and typically attached to products making false claims such as those popular metabolism booster supplements. It's especially important for people trying to gain better control of their weight to understand the intertwined concepts of metabolism, energy, and weight loss.

The first equations that you must understand and that are essential to guiding you successfully to your weight loss goals are centered around energy.

energy in = energy out
    or
energy consumed = energy expended

If you can maintain this balanced state between the energy you put into your body and the energy that your body expends, then at the very least you'll maintain your current weight. What happens when you consume more energy than you expend?

energy in > energy out = weight gain

If you consume more food energy than your body needs or is able to burn off, then that excess energy gets stored as fat and results in weight gain.

You can, however, lose weight by manipulating the second half of the equation.

ENERGY IN < ENERGY OUT = WEIGHT LOSS

If your body burns off more energy than it consumes, it must get this energy from somewhere. That's where your energy-rich fat takes a leading role. Now you can kill two birds with one stone. Not only are you able to meet your body's energy requirement, but you're also able to lose excess fat. Now the rest of the reasoning becomes simple. The greater the difference between the energy consumed and the energy expended, the greater the amount of fat you can burn, thus the greater the weight loss.

So where does metabolism fit into all of this? Metabolism does its work on the right side of the equation. There are two major ways through which the body burns or expends energy—metabolism and physical activities. We'll discuss the energy cost of physical activities in a later chapter, but for now we'll focus on how your metabolism plays a key role in the amount of weight you gain and how fast or slowly you can lose it.

There are several involuntary activities that you participate in during the course of the day without even thinking about them. Blood circulation, breathing, body temperature maintenance, hormone secretion, nerve activity, and new tissue synthesis are just a few of the many activities that occur around the clock without your conscious or direct control. The sum of all of these activities is called "basal metabolism," and the rate at which the body uses energy to support them is called the "basal metabolic rate" (BMR). No two people are the same, and thus our BMRs can vary as widely as the color and texture of our hair or skin.

Your BMR can be an essential determinant of whether your body will gain or lose weight, because it constitutes approximately 60–65 percent of your daily energy expenditure, making it the body's greatest way of expending energy. BMR is followed by the energy expenditure of physical activity (approximatimately 25–35 percent) and the energy consumed while digesting food (about 5–10 percent). The bad news, especially for dieters, is that the major factors that influence your BMR are largely out of your control. The older you get, the slower your BMR, largely because your lean body mass (muscle-to-fat ratio) declines as you age. The taller you are, the higher your BMR, because you have more surface area, which requires more energy to maintain. Children and pregnant women typically have higher BMRs because they're in a rapid growth phase. Fever and stress, two conditions that aren't typically favorable to your overall health, actually increase your BMR. Those who think that fasting or starving will help them lose weight are only half right. You certainly will drop significant weight in the beginning of a fast, but during this period, the body responds by trying to conserve energy rather than expending it, so it automatically lowers your BMR. This is why people who go on fasting diets reach a plateau after a certain amount of weight loss and can't seem to get over it. The hormone thyroxine, produced by the thyroid gland, is an important regulator of your BMR. The more you produce—as in people with the medical condition hyperthyroidism—the higher your BMR. The converse is also true, as demonstrated in patients who are hypothyroid, or have an underactive thyroid gland. Their metabolism slows down, which tips the energy equation to the left and results in weight gain. This, of course, can be overcome by increasing physical activity to a high enough level that it also increases total energy expenditure.

People are constantly asking me about the effectiveness of these metabolism boosters that are featured in TV advertisements and glossy magazines. The simple truth is that there's no safe and effective way to boost your metabolism to the levels it would require to induce significant weight loss. These processes that make up metabolism are largely unresponsive to external influences, unless you consume one of the compounds that has thyroxine-like effects or increases the activities of the autonomic nervous system. Not only are these supplements largely unregulated by the federal government, but they can cause serious damage that extends far beyond the potential benefits of weight loss.

CHAPTER 7

AIM FOR THE RIGHT TARGET

Your Weight Loss Goals

The word *fat* can conjure up depressing and even painful associations for many people. The negative images associated with being overweight are constantly pounded into our subconscious, so much so that we automatically adopt the attached societal stigmas. There are people who have been overweight since childhood and have lived with the constant reminders of their excessive weight, whether through derisive comments made by others or the feelings of being ostracized by others who judge them not by what's on the inside, but by their physical appearance.

IN DEFENSE OF FAT

Despite all its negative connotations, fat is actually an essential part of our bodies, a component without which we wouldn't be able to live. At the most fundamental biological level, fat plays an extremely important role in the membrane or outer covering of our cells. Each cell contains these lipid structures that regulate what enters and exits the cell. These fatty elements are conveniently constructed out of the many different foods we eat.

The fats in our foods and bodies, otherwise known as lipids, fall into three major classes: triglycerides (about 95 percent of all lipids, the major storage form of fat, and what we usually mean when we say fat), phospholipids, and sterols (cholesterol is the best-known example). Our most immediate and important demand of fats is the energy that they can provide. For each gram of fat, your body can harvest 9 calories of energy. This energy from fat can, of course, work both ways. While fat is an excellent source of energy that the body utilizes when other more immediate forms are not available, if we consume more fat energy in our diets than we actually need or are able to burn through physical activity or metabolism, the excess will be stored in our adipose tissue (fat cells).

Each person is born with approximately the number of fat cells that they will have for the rest of their lives—about three billion. The body stores excess energy by packing the triglycerides into these fat cells. Our ability to store fat is essentially limitless; in fact, one fat cell can increase about fifty times its original weight. If the cells in our bodies are filled to capacity and we continue to consume more energy than we expend, our bodies simply form new adipose cells.

Beyond providing the body with emergency energy, fat is important for its protective purposes. It surrounds vital organs, serving as a shock absorber when the body is suddenly jostled or experiences excessive movements. Fat allows us to ride a horse for an extended period of time or ride inside an off-road vehicle on bumpy terrain without suffering internal injuries. Fat helps regulate our internal temperature, keeping us warm when the outside temperature is very cold or keeping us from overheating when the ambient temperature is extremely hot. We take for granted the number of times we sit down during the course of the day without injuring our bones. These comfortable landings are due to the blanket of fat pads that insulate our muscles and bones.

THE CALCULATOR: DETERMINING HOW MUCH FAT YOU NEED TO LOSE

For many people, what they *actually* weigh can be quite different from what they *think* they weigh. Our self-perceptions of weight can be influenced by several factors, including the opinions others have of us, how we prefer to look, and the appearance of others around us. Weight and appearance are tightly woven into our self-image, which often leads to distorted claims about being overweight, of normal weight, or too thin. It's important to know your true dimensions, because they can be used to determine whether or not you fall into a healthy weight range. For the last fifty years, doctors and other health professionals have used weight-for-height tables issued by the Metropolitan Life Insurance Company. These tables consider your gender, body frame, and height and, through a population average, show you what would be considered an ideal weight range.

These tables are still used, but they've fallen out of favor in recent years, not because they are defective, but because newer measurement techniques have been shown to be more effective at determining body fat content. Now the most widely accepted measurement is the body mass index (BMI). This is defined as the average relative weight for height in people older than twenty years, and it usually correlates with body fatness and degree of disease risks associated with being overweight or underweight. BMI can be calculated easily if you know your height and weight.

$$BMI = \frac{\text{weight (kg)}}{\text{height (m) x height (m)}}$$

or

$$BMI = \frac{\text{weight (lb.) x 705}}{\text{height (in.) x height (in.)}}$$

Here's how I calculate my BMI:

Height: 6 feet 2 inches = 74 inches
Weight: 185 pounds
So, $\frac{185 \text{ (lb.) x } 705}{74 \text{ in. x } 74 \text{ in.}} = 23.8$

The following table explains the different BMI measurements and their classification:

BMI	OBESITY CLASS	RISKS TO HEALTH
<18.5	Underweight	Lower the BMI, greater the risk
18.5 through 24.9	Normal	Very low risk
25.0 through 29.9	Overweight	Increased risk/high risk

BMI	OBESITY CLASS	RISKS TO HEALTH
30.0 through 34.9	Class I obesity	High risk/very high risk
35.0 through 39.9	Class II obesity	Very high risk
40.0 or above	Class III obesity	Extreme risk

Source: Sizer and Whitney, *Nutrition: Concepts and Controversies*, 8th ed. (New York: Wadsworth Thomson Learning, Belmont, CA) 2000.

While BMI is one of the most accurate measurements for evaluating degrees of fatness in those who are overweight or obese, it's less accurate in those considered to be nonobese. Two of the major drawbacks of BMI are that it fails to indicate how much of the weight is fat and where that fat is located. You can imagine a couple of situations in which the BMI wouldn't be accurate in measuring the body mass index. Athletes who are in great shape and have large muscles can have a falsely reported BMI, because their weight might be increased, but this weight is mostly muscle and not fat. Pregnant and lactating women would also have deceptively elevated BMIs, and this would be expected because of the necessary increase in weight gain during normal childbearing. Adults over sixty-five might also have BMIs that aren't truly indicative of their degree of fatness, because the BMI chart values that are used have been based on data collected from younger people. Also, it's not surprising that as we age, our height diminishes, which could also alter the measurement.

Those for whom the BMI isn't an accurate measure for the reasons stated above should use a standard height and weight chart like the one that follows or consult with their physicians, who can make a more accurate assessment.

HEIGHT-WEIGHT CHART

WOMEN (Pounds)

HEIGHT	SMALL FRAME	MEDIUM FRAME	LARGE FRAME
4'10"	102–111	109–121	118–131
4'11"	103–113	111–123	120–134

HEIGHT	SMALL FRAME	MEDIUM FRAME	LARGE FRAME
5'0"	104–115	113–126	122–137
5'1"	106–118	115–129	125–140
5'2"	108–121	118–132	128–143
5'3"	111–124	121–135	131–147
5'4"	114–127	124–138	134–151
5'5"	117–130	127–141	137–155
5'6"	120–133	130–144	140–159
5'7"	123–136	133–147	143–163
5'8"	126–139	136–150	146–167
5'9"	129–142	139–153	149–170
5'10"	132–145	142–156	152–173
5'11"	135–148	145–159	155–176
6'0"	138–151	148–162	158–179

MEN (Pounds)

HEIGHT	SMALL FRAME	MEDIUM FRAME	LARGE FRAME
5'2"	128–134	131–141	138–150
5'3"	130–136	133–143	140–153
5'4"	132–138	135–145	142–156
5'5"	134–140	137–148	144–160
5'6"	136–142	139–151	146–164
5'7"	138–145	142–154	149–168
5'8"	140–148	145–157	152–172
5'9"	142–151	148–160	155–176
5'10"	144–154	151–163	158–180
5'11"	146–157	154–166	161–184
6'0"	149–160	157–170	164–188
6'1"	152–164	160–174	168–192
6'2"	155–168	164–178	172–197

HEIGHT	SMALL FRAME	MEDIUM FRAME	LARGE FRAME
6'3"	158–172	167–182	176–202
6'4"	162–176	171–187	181–207

From Metropolitan Life Insurance. The Metropolitan Life Insuance Company devised this chart based on the weights of people who lived the longest in each height category.

How to lose the fat and keep the muscle in a healthy, long-lasting way is the subject of the next several chapters.

PART FOUR

BE IN CHARGE OF THE FEAST

CHAPTER 8

REAL FOOD

Eating More for Less

Over a period of a couple of months, I noticed that one of my colleagues had lost a considerable amount of weight. In fact, her clothes were beginning to hang off her, clearly indicating they were too large for her trimmed frame. I finally asked how she had been able to lose so much weight. "I've stopped eating bread and sweets," she answered proudly. "I've lost twenty-five pounds and have never felt better. I'm determined to keep it off." She went on to describe her low-carbohydrate diet, which meant severely restricting her consumption of carbs, particularly in the form of sweets such as cookies, cake, and soda.

After hearing her explanation, I asked about her level of exercise. I was most interested in learning whether or not she had been boosting the effects of a lower-calorie diet by simultaneously increasing her level of physical activity.

"That's the amazing thing," she said, and laughed. "I haven't been to the gym once and I lost all of this weight. I can't stand the gym."

You can probably imagine my internal natural urges begging me to explain to her the importance of exercise and physical activity in any weight loss program, but I decided not to dampen her spirits. I just listened, knowing that it was going to be almost impossible for her to keep this weight off without an activity program, especially since she had lost the weight on a diet that would be nearly impossible to stick to.

A few weeks after the initial conversation with my colleague, I noticed that her clothes were not as baggy as they had been over the past several weeks. She had either bought a new wardrobe or the weight had returned. She came clean on her own.

"I couldn't take it," she confessed. "It was fine for a couple of months, but eating everything without bread and not eating chocolate was impossible. I don't know who can stick to that kind of diet. It's not normal."

The truth of the matter is that very few people can survive these severely restrictive diets. We simply don't form our eating habits overnight; rather, they are the results of choices made over the course of a lifetime. You can't expect that after thirty years of eating your hot dog on a bun you can suddenly stop and eat it off the plate for the rest of your life. Your sense of taste isn't accustomed to eating hot dogs that way, and it will tell you that you find the hot dog not as appetizing as it used to be. Most dieters will, in fact, admit that the programs they've found the most success on are not those that require the severe restriction or total elimination of certain foods. Instead, those diets that only limit the intake of certain high-calorie foods and suggest a plan of physical activity appear to be most likely to provide some long-term weight loss.

First, list the top ten foods that you can never seem to get enough of and review them for their calorie and fat content. I did this myself and found that at the top of my list were french fries, bacon, and chocolate-chip cookies. I spent one whole week reviewing what I ate and found that every day I had an order of fries, whether it was with lunch or dinner. When I went grocery shopping, I always threw a couple of bags of chocolate-chip cookies in the cart and filled the cookie jar at home. Throughout the day, even first thing in the morning, I found myself going to the cookie jar and grabbing two or three at a time, easily emptying the jar in a week's time. I finally decided that as much as I liked my fries and cookies, if I limited my consumption, I would not only keep off the extra weight, but I could substitute other foods such as fruits and vegetables. These substitutions would still take the sting off the between meals hunger pangs, but with fewer calories and more nutritional offerings such as vitamins and minerals.

SATIETY: HOW THE BODY RESPONDS TO HUNGER

Much research has gone into understanding what happens when the body sends signals to the brain that it's hungry and how the eating response helps to satisfy this hunger. At some point during a meal, the brain is flooded with nerve and chemical signals that send a message that enough food has been eaten. This condition of fullness and communication to the brain is called satiation. It's a most important process to monitor in hopes of preventing overeating and weight gain.

Eliminating the desire to eat is more complicated than simply eating a meal. Eating in response to hunger will lead to a feeling of satisfaction, but there are a number of steps in between the act of eating and the brain sending back signals that no more food needs to be eaten. The hypothalamus, a portion of the brain that's believed to serve several functions, from regulating our body temperature to influencing the development of secondary sex characteristics, plays a critical role in the regulation of satiety. Once a certain group of cells in the feeding centers of the hypothalamus are stimulated, they signal us to eat. Our hunger is decreased as we respond by eating. The process of eating stimulates another group of cells located in the satiety centers of the hypothalamus, cells that eventually send signals to stop eating. Several experiments have been conducted that destroy the hypothalamic satiety centers in lab animals. The result: these animals don't receive the proper impulses to stop eating when the hunger has been satisfied, and they munch their way to obesity.

One of the most important factors that influences satiety is the size of a meal. When food stretches our stomachs, signals are sent via nerves to the brain communicating how much has been eaten and how much of the stomach capacity has been filled. The meal is broken down by a series of enzymes, starting first in the stomach and then in the intestines as the meal continues to make its way down the GI tract. Special cells line the entire tract, and their major responsibility is the absorption of nutrients and other products of food metabolism. As these cells carry out their absorption duties, they send special signals to the brain indicating that a meal has been eaten and it's time to start shutting down the hunger drive to consume more food.

It takes your body about twenty minutes to send a signal to your brain that your hunger has been appeased. For this reason, eating slowly will greatly help you keep from overeating and from feeling deprived or hungry after a meal.

ENERGY DENSITY OF FOODS

The three most important aspects of food are taste, the amount of energy it contains, and the nutritional content. Taste, of course, is often an individual perception, which among other variables helps determine our preference for certain foods. The amount of energy packed into a certain food, however, remains constant regardless of how much the food appeals to us or how much of it we eat. The fancy name for a food's energy content is called the energy density (ED):

> **ENERGY DENSITY:** The number of calories contained within 1 gram of a particular food.

Like most things related to science, the concept is much simpler than it sounds. Imagine five identical cars weighing the same as they come off the assembly line. However, as people sit inside, the weight changes. The more people in the car, the more dense the car becomes. You can apply this analogy to foods. Though fat, alcohol, carbohydrate, protein, and water don't look alike, the calories they contain are similar to the people getting into the car. Fat packs in the most people, or calories, at 9. Alcohol has an energy density of 7. Carbohydrate and protein contain only 4 calories. Water, regardless of how much, packs no energy; therefore its energy density is 0. There's a simple way to calculate a food's energy density:

$$\text{energy density} = \frac{\text{\# calories}}{1 \text{ gram}}$$

For example, take a look at the back of a bag of Fritos.

Nutrition Facts
Serving Size 1 oz. (28g/About 32 chips)
Servings Per Container 4.5

Amount Per Serving	
Calories 160	Calories from Fat 90

To calculate the energy density, you would use the equation above and divide 160 calories by 28 grams. This delivers an ED of 5.7. Compare this to what you'd get from a can of small whole carrots.

Nutrition Facts

Serving Size ½ cup (123 g)
Servings Per Container about 2

Amount Per Serving	
Calories 30	Calories from Fat 0

The ED from this can of carrots is calculated by dividing 30 calories by 123 grams. This delivers an ED of 0.24. As you can see, if you were to eat the same weight (grams) of Fritos as these canned carrots, the Fritos would pack approximately twenty-four more times the amount of energy (5.7 divided by 0.24 = 23.75). Researchers from Penn State have done an extensive amount of research on the energy density of foods and how they factor into our weight management. They have conveniently divided the food groups according to their energy densities, as follows:

CATEGORY 1: VERY LOW-ENERGY-DENSE FOODS   ED less than 0.6: includes most fruits and vegetables, skim milk, and broth-based soups.

CATEGORY 2: LOW-ENERGY-DENSE FOODS   ED 0.6–1.5: includes many cooked grains, breakfast cereals with low-fat milk, low-fat meats, beans and legumes, low-fat mixed dishes, and salads.

CATEGORY 3: MEDIUM-ENERGY-DENSE FOODS   ED 1.5–4.0: includes meats, cheeses, high-fat mixed dishes, salad dressings, poultry, and some snack foods.

CATEGORY 4: HIGH-ENERGY-DENSE FOODS   ED 4.0–9.0: includes crackers, chips, chocolate candies, cookies, nuts, butter, and full-fat condiments.*

*Source: Rolls and Barnett, *Volumetrics* (New York: HarperCollins), 2000, p. 15.

So when you get that between meal urge to snack, reaching for a bag of Fritos means that you're choosing a high ED food. If, instead, you had a small can's worth of carrots that you kept conveniently nearby, you'd be choosing a very low ED food. Research has repeatedly shown that our sense of satisfaction is determined by the volume of food we eat, not the type. Whether you're eating half a pound of cherries or half a pound of meat, both theoretically will fill you up the same. However, as you can imagine, the cherries would have a much lower ED, which means you're still satisfying your hunger, but with less energy— perfect for our plan to reduce energy consumption. In the appendix (see page 184), you'll find a table listing the energy densities of over six hundred foods.

Understanding the energy density concept can be valuable when taking control of your dietary choices. If you can't sit down and calculate the exact energy densities of the foods you're about to eat, you can at least have some idea by looking at the table provided in the appendix. You can also think about which foods might have a higher water content. Remember, water has an ED of 0, so the more water a food contains, the lower the ED. For instance, look at the example of apples versus dried apple slices. A normal fresh apple with the peel and measuring 3¼ inches in diameter contains 81 calories. However, if you wanted to eat the equivalent amount of calories in dried apple slices, you'd be able to eat only six slices. The apple weighs in at 212 grams, while the six dried slices weigh 38.4 grams. If you were to eat equivalent volumes to satisfy your hunger (remember, volume is what fills us up), you'd have to eat thirty-three slices of dried apples. This, of course, would be disastrous for our attempts to reduce energy consumption.

APPLE	DRIED APPLE CHIPS IN A BOWL
212 gm	212 gm
81 cal.	514 cal.

You can choose either one to help relieve those hunger pangs, but if you choose the fresh apple, you'll obviously be making the wiser energy choice. The heavy water content of the apple gives it great volume at little energy cost, because water has an ED of 0. Part of your strategy in selecting less fattening foods should obviously include skipping those foods that have lots of calories packed into small volumes and choosing those that have a higher content of water. "Energy Density Spectrum for Selected Foods" (see appendix, page 184) lists the energy densities of common foods.

FATS: THE GOOD, THE BAD, AND THE UGLY

As ironic as it might sound in the midst of today's "fat-free" hysteria, fat is also important in our diets, because it brings along with it a certain set of vitamins called the "fat-soluble" vitamins. These essential nutrients are dissolved in fat and include the vitamins A, D, E, and K. One of the major reasons we don't often run deficient in these vitamins is that the body has the ability to store them in our fat cells. Other vitamins are water-soluble, so once the body has met its demand for them, the surplus is excreted. Foods rich in these vitamins must be ingested constantly to meet the necessary requirements.

It's no accident that we like to consume foods with higher concentrations of fat. Our evolutionary memory desires fat as protection against starvation, and as a result we are genetically programmed to crave fatty foods. Fat carries with it many dissolved compounds that release those enticing aromas, such as frying bacon, that you can smell across the room. Fat also has a texture and an array of flavors that your mouth, stomach, and brain aren't soon to forget. Fat can also add to the tenderness of meats and baked goods, making these foods easy to eat.

SATURATED VERSUS UNSATURATED FATS

How many times have you read or heard the term *saturated fatty acid* and shaken your head in confusion? Until I went to medical school, I had the same reaction. When people started talking about saturated versus polyunsaturated fats, they might as well have been speaking another language. However, once you get a basic understanding of these concepts, you realize why health experts make such a big fuss over these terms.

The word *saturation* refers to the number of hydrogens a fatty acid chain is holding. If the fatty acid contains the largest number of hydrogen atoms as possible, the fat is saturated (literally *filled*). When there are points along the chain where a hydrogen is missing, this is called a point of unsaturation and the fat is classified as unsaturated. If there's only one point, it's a monounsaturated fatty acid, but if there's more than one point, it's called a polyunsaturated fatty acid.

These little hydrogen atoms and their effects on the different fatty acids are of enormous consequence. Several studies have shown that the more saturated the fat, the greater your increased risk for heart disease. Conversely, the less the fatty chain is saturated with hydrogen, the lower your risk for elevated cholesterol levels and cardiovascular-related problems such as heart attack and stroke.

Saturated fats increase one's risk of heart disease because they raise blood cholesterol. It follows that foods rich in both saturated fat and cholesterol can cause problems for people attempting to lower blood cholesterol. Saturated fats are usually solid at room temperature. They are commonly found in meat and poultry, as well as whole-milk dairy products such as cheese, milk, ice cream, cream, butter, and lard.

Monounsaturated fats are liquid at room temperature but start to solidify at refrigerator temperatures. Salad dressing that contains olive oil is a good example. When it's in the refrigerator, it's cloudy, but when it's left out for a while, it's clear. It's believed that these fats actually lower blood cholesterol.

Polyunsaturated fatty acids are liquid at room temperature and in the refrigerator. You might recognize them by the sometimes rancid smell that emanates from the fats as they combine with oxygen. Vegetable oils and oils derived from seeds are examples of polyunsaturated fats. Polyunsaturated fats actually help lower total blood cholesterol.

Trans-fatty acids contain a combination of the three types of fats and similar carbon and hydrogen atoms as the other fats, but they are arranged in a completely different order. Trans-fatty acids occur in nature as the result of fermentation in grazing animals. People eat them in the form of meat and dairy products. Trans-fatty acids are also formed through a particular chemical process—hydrogenation—used to give texture to certain vegetable or fish oils. Hydrogenating polyunsaturated oils allows foods to stay fresh on the shelf, and they solidify fat products such as margarine, so that they don't melt at room temperature. Popular foods such as cookies, crackers, and pastries can have a large amount of trans-fats,—yet another reason why you want to eat them in moderation, especially if you already have other heart disease risk factors.

While adding hydrogen to these oils has its uses, health advocates are very concerned about its potential hazards. Several clinical studies have shown that trans-fatty acids raise the "bad" LDL cholesterol while lowering the "good" HDL cholesterol. This alteration in cholesterol composition can predispose people to heart disease, which is why several health organizations, including the American Heart Association, have warned people to be careful of how much of these particular fats they consume. One study out of the Netherlands showed that people who consumed a higher diet of trans-fats had a 29 percent reduction in blood vessel function and a lowering of HDL cholesterol by 20 percent. There are no standard methods to estimate the trans-fatty acid content of food, and some labels don't even include it in their lists of ingredients. There is one tip, however, you can use when searching the food label—look for the words *hydrogenated oils.*

Olive oil is by far one of the most popular oils around, used frequently in salad dressing and as a dipping condiment for bread. It has gotten a lot of attention from the media lately because several studies have shown that people who eat a diet that includes olive oil and other unsaturated fats have a marked reduction in risk for heart disease. People who consume diets high in unsaturated fat and low in saturated fat also tend to have lower blood pressure. Although olive oil displays these benefits, it is still a fat and when eaten in excessive amounts can override the health benefits of moderate consumption.

You can typically tell what type of fat a food contains by reading the food label, but that's not the only way. Looking at the hardness of the fat can be another important clue. How much a fatty acid is saturated affects the temperature at which the fat melts. Basically, the more unsaturated the fatty acid, the more liquid a fat will be standing at room temperature. If you're trying to determine whether an oil you use contains saturated fats, you can place the oil in a clear container in the refrigerator and watch how cloudy it becomes. The most unsaturated oils remain the clearest.

As a general rule of thumb, vegetable and fish oils are rich in polyunsaturated fats. Some vegetable oils, such as olive oil, are also rich in monounsaturated fats. Animal fats tend to be the most saturated. Choosing a plant oil, however, doesn't always mean that you're choosing the heart-healthy polyunsaturated oils. Coconut oil, for example, comes from a plant, but it disobeys the general rule that plant oils are less saturated than animal fats. In fact, coconut oil is severely more saturated and contributes to heart disease risk. Palm oil, a one-time common oil used in frying foods, has also been added to the list of oils that increase your cholesterol levels and heart disease risk because of its highly saturated structure.

FIBER—YOUR WEIGHT LOSS ALLY

Out of the hundreds of lectures that I sat through in medical school, I can't remember one dedicated to nutritional fiber and its effects on the body. Nutrition isn't a widely taught course in medical school, which seems odd since physicians must treat all types of problems, including nutritional deficiencies. I became particularly interested in nutrition when friends and family members would ask me questions about their food choices and what effects they had on the body.

Fiber is one of those nutritional topics that mysteriously gets less than its share of attention. Most people probably don't know that fiber is considered to be a carbohydrate just like sugars and starch. It's the part of whole grains, vegetables, fruits, and nuts that resists digestion in the gastrointestinal tract. Most fibers are chains of sugars held together by bonds that human digestive enzymes can't break. Some fibers are soluble in water, whereas others are not, and typically, foods contain a combination. You've been looking at fiber all of your life but didn't realize it: fiber helps form the supporting structures of a plant, including its leaves, stems, and seeds. The best-known fibers are cellulose, hemicellulose, and pectin, which are commonly found in the strands of celery, skins of corn kernels, and membranes surrounding kernels of wheat. Pectin is found in apples and citrus fruits and is also used to thicken jelly and other processed foods. When your doctor recommends that you increase the "roughage" in your diet, he or she is usually referring to these fibers.

Dietary fibers have numerous functions in the body; most notably they promote feelings of fullness. Fiber has a great proclivity to absorb surrounding water in the gastrointestinal tract and swell. When a sufficient amount of fiber has been consumed, its ability to absorb and retain water helps enlarge and soften the stool, making elimination easier. When not enough fiber is eaten, as is quite common in the United States, it has the opposite effect on the stool, making it hard and compact. This, unfortunately, leads to constipation, where the intestine has a difficult time expelling the stool. Thus, when people (especially older people) experience continuous bouts of constipation, doctors will often recommend increasing their dietary fiber.

One of fiber's various functions that has gotten a lot of press in the last couple of years has been its possible role in preventing colon and rectal cancers. Researchers haven't yet reached a unanimous decision on fiber's ability to prevent these intestinal cancers, but several epidemiological studies have drawn global interest to this possibility.

Epidemiologists have looked at the link between colon cancer and dietary habits and found that diets low in whole grains, fruits, and vegetables are linked to a higher incidence of cancer. These foods, of course, are excellent sources of fiber, which has many researchers thinking it's the lack of dietary fiber that could be the problem.

A 1992 study by researchers at Harvard Medical School found that men who consumed 12 grams of fiber a day were twice as likely to develop precancerous colon changes as men whose daily fiber intake was about 30 grams. The confusing issue for most consumers is that for virtually every study that shows the great promise of fiber in cancer prevention, there's a study that demonstrates little or no effect at all.

Many researchers instead point to other factors that seem to make a greater contribution, including genetic background and inflammatory diseases of the intestine.

Cardiologists also sing the praises of fiber, especially in light of the numerous studies that suggest increased dietary fiber levels can actually decrease levels of blood cholesterol. According to the Food and Drug Administration (FDA), clinical studies show that cholesterol levels dropped between 0.5 percent and 2 percent for every gram of soluble fiber eaten per day. It's believed that as soluble fiber passes through the GI tract, it binds to dietary cholesterol and helps the body eliminate it.

Fiber can also protect against heart attacks. Two long-term large-scale studies of men suggest that high fiber intake can significantly lower the risk for heart attack. In the U.S. study of more than forty-three thousand male health professionals, those who ate more than 25 grams of fiber per day had a 36 percent lower risk for developing heart disease than those who consumed less than 15 grams daily. In a Finnish study, each 10 grams of fiber added to the diet decreased the risk of dying from heart disease by 17 percent. This benefit was even greater in the U.S. study, where the risk reduction was shown to be decreased by 29 percent.

Adequate fiber consumption has even been linked to helping diabetics better handle their blood sugar. Fiber's ability to slow the absorption of glucose from the small intestine has made it a potential diabetes fighter. A study from the Harvard School of Public Health and published in the *Journal of the American Medical Association* suggests that a high-sugar, low-fiber diet more than doubles a woman's risk for type II diabetes. This study found that cereal fiber was associated with a 28 percent decreased risk. (Interestingly, fruit and vegetable fiber had no effect on the risk of diabetes. That, however, does not negate their overall fiber value with regard to dieting.) Increased consumption of cola beverages, white bread, white rice, and french fries elevated the risk.

By now you're probably wondering about fiber's role in promoting weight loss. The first advantage that fiber provides is its ability to make you feel fuller for a longer period of time. High-fiber foods typically take longer to chew, and because fiber absorbs water, it provides bulk to the diet and promotes the feeling of fullness. The water-soluble fiber found in fruits, legumes, seeds, and oat products exit the stomach more slowly, which also helps you feel full longer.

Fiber itself contains no calories and is typically found in foods that are also low-fat (fruits, vegetables, whole grains, breads, and cereals). Eating diets higher in fiber often means consuming less calories; the foods themselves don't contain many calories, and there's not much room left to eat fattening foods because the fiber-containing foods fill most of the stomach. Fiber might also reduce the available energy from other foods, most notably calorie-dense dietary fat. It's also believed to help sustain higher energy levels, reducing hunger pangs between meals.

For all of its observed and potential benefits, surprisingly, most Americans don't eat anywhere near the amount of fiber that professional health organizations recommend. According to the third National Health and Nutritional Survey, the average fiber consumption here in the United States is approximately 14–15 grams per day. This falls far below the 25–30 grams per day recommended by the American Dietetic Association and the 20–30 grams recommended by the National Cancer Institute. Epidemiologists have studied the dietary fiber intake trends in the United States and compared them to trends in other parts of the world, such as Asia and Africa, whose populations eat diets higher in fruits and vegetables. They've found an amazing difference in many diseases believed to be prevented by fiber, most notably colon diseases such as polyps, diverticulitis, and colon cancer.

Despite fiber's potential benefits, it's important to increase fiber in your diet slowly. This gives you time to build a tolerance and avoid the cramping and bloating that can accompany large amounts of dietary fiber. Most at risk are those who quickly add a great deal of dietary fiber—for example, 60 grams per day—without making the necessary adjustments in their diets. It's important to consume plenty of water and other caffeine-free fluids, since fiber absorbs water. Maintaining an adequate intake of vitamins and minerals is also important, as extremely high amounts of fiber can deplete them from the body, especially calcium, zinc, and iron. (See appendix, "Recommended Dietary Intakes," page 197.) While fibers are an important part of the diet, not all fiber-based products are safe; in fact, some can even prove to be harmful. For example, the FDA has taken legal action against several fiber-based products containing guar gum, which has been linked to obstructions in the intestines, stomach, and esophagus.

Here are some tips on increasing your fiber consumption:

EAT MORE LEGUMES Beans are rich in fiber, contain high-quality protein, and are low in dietary fat.

INCREASE VEGETABLE CONSUMPTION Corn, tomatoes, cabbage,

broccoli, cauliflower, green beans, and zucchini are all loaded with fiber.

ADD MORE FRUIT TO YOUR DIET Try more bananas, grapes, peaches, apricots, and strawberries. They're full of fiber.

EAT HIGH-FIBER CEREALS Simply by reading the food nutrition label, you'll be able to identify those cereals high in fiber.

OPT FOR BROWN RICE It contains more fiber than white rice.

GO NUTTY As long as you don't have allergies, chomp on more nuts. They're full of insoluble fiber.

WHOLE-GRAIN EXTRAVAGANZA Whole-grain bread and wheat bran are excellent fiber sources.

BERRY BERRY GOOD Add them to your pancake and waffle mix or muffin batter.

When deciding what foods are right for your diet, giving thoughtful consideration to increasing the fiber content to 30–35 grams can be important to your health and your efforts to lose weight. "Fiber Content of Foods" (see appendix, page 188), compiled by Tufts University School of Medicine, will help you become familiar with high-fiber foods that you should include in your diet.

THE GLYCEMIC INDEX OF FOODS

With all the talk of low-carbohydrate diets and the negative consequences of excess sugar consumption, it's important to give some attention to how different foods can affect the body's chemistry, particularly the hormone insulin. Insulin is secreted by the pancreas into the blood. Its major function is to help transport glucose from the blood into the cells. Once the cells have absorbed the glucose, they can break it down and use it for energy or store it in the liver or muscles as glycogen, which can be released later when the body's energy demands increase.

How fast the carbohydrate load of a particular food is converted to glucose and enters the blood is called "the glycemic index" (GI). The speed with which blood sugar levels rise is given a number that's a percentage of what's considered to be a reference food—typically, white bread. The references are assigned a value of 100, and everything else is a percentage of that. For example, the glycemic index of an oatmeal cookie is 78, whereas the GI of peanuts is only 15. However, there are some types of food that make the blood sugar level rise faster than if one had eaten white bread. These foods have a GI greater than 100 and include instant boiled rice at 121 and baked potatoes at 128.

Why does all of this matter? At the center of some diets is the belief that the most concerning aspect about eating is the glycemic index. They postulate that high-glycemic foods are more likely to increase body fat by increasing the amount of insulin that's secreted and causing a rapid absorption of glucose from the blood that gets stored as fat. Most scientists will agree that the glycemic index does exist, but that's as far as the agreement goes. In fact, there's a large controversy about whether the glycemic index really has any direct relationship to weight gain and obesity. Many of these diet books would have you believe that simply choosing foods that have a low glycemic index will result in your ability to prevent weight gain. But the obesity experts continue to explain that obesity isn't about the rate at which glucose rises in the blood, it's the number of calories that are actually consumed.

Another problem with relying on the glycemic index as a way to determine the food choices you make is that having a low GI doesn't necessarily mean a food is healthful or low in calories. For example, a ½ cup serving of Ben & Jerry's rich vanilla ice cream has a GI of 52 but contains 230 calories. Compare this to an equal weight (in grams) of cooked carrots, which have a GI of 117 but contain only 48 calories. It's ridiculous, of course, to suggest that someone should eat more ice cream than carrots, simply because the ice cream has a lower GI, when in reality it has more than four times the number of calories for a given serving. This is why many weight experts insist that the glycemic index is an interesting phenomenon and possibly more applicable to diabetics, who typically are unable to control their blood sugar levels and thus are at more risk with foods that increase these levels dramatically and quickly. Even for those who are not diabetic, consuming foods with a high GI can cause rapid energy fluctuations that result in energy "crashes." The best approach is to eat a variety of foods at each meal.

Another flaw in the glycemic index theory of weight loss is that when we eat meals, they are typically mixed. Most people, for example, don't have just a plate of fries or a bowl of tortilla chips. When the foods are well balanced with meats, starches, and vegetables, a part of the meal will have a high GI, while another part will fall into the low GI category. This combination will lessen the effect of the GI on the body's internal chemistry, not causing the blood sugars to rise as when eating just one high GI food by itself. Stick to counting calories and increasing your physical activity—most experts agree that this is the best way to prevent weight gain and to shrink those stubborn pockets of fat.

The appendix includes a glycemic index table for selected foods (see page 191).

CAN FOODS AFFECT YOUR METABOLISM?

A popular belief among many dieters is that certain foods can actually increase your metabolism. I've heard that everything from a diet based on grapefruit to one full of cabbage soup can help boost your metabolism and help burn away the fat. This sounds like a great idea: simply choose a certain group of foods and watch the fat melt away without the need to count your calories or exercise. The truth, however, falls far away from these enthusiastic claims.

There is something called the thermogenic effect of food, in which just the act of digesting food is a certain amount of work that requires calories. It's believed that this process of thermogenesis accounts for 5–10 percent of all the energy we expend in the course of the day. Different nutrients do require different amounts of work to complete the digestion of foods, with pure protein using the most energy. High-fiber complex carbohydrates are next, requiring more energy to digest than fats and refined sugars. Some diet programs have tried to capitalize on this difference in digestive energy requirements by suggesting a diet high in lean protein and high-fiber complex carbohydrates and limiting the amount of foods made from refined flours and sugars.

It's true that these nutrients will help increase your digestive energy demand, and thus your metabolism, but what many of these dieting programs don't tell you is that this effect is only temporary, typically peaking within an hour after eating. The amount that these foods raise your metabolism is minimal, certainly not enough to suggest that making major dietary changes will be a tremendous help in shedding those excess pounds.

GENERAL GUIDELINES

The USDA's Food Guide Pyramid is an excellent nutritional guideline. Decades of research both in the physiology of nutrition and people's eating patterns have helped form the USDA's dietary guidelines. The USDA uses information from several sources, including leading health and nutrition scientists from around the country and the world, to form these dietary recommendations. According to the USDA's dietary guidelines for Americans, our diets should consist of 55–65 percent carbohydrate, 20–30 percent fat, and 10–15 percent protein. These are only recommendations and not hard and fast rules, so there's a little room to individualize these percentages. The appendix offers the USDA Food Guide Pyramid and also details the USDA's recommended dietary intakes (see pages 194 and 197).

CHAPTER 9

HAVE IT YOUR WAY

Menus for a Healthier You

N ow that you know what a calorie actually is and you understand the most important concept in weight loss—energy in must be less than energy out—it's time to take control of your diet and start shedding those pounds. Remember that this isn't a gimmick where you blindly adhere to a strange regimen of low carbs and high protein or vice versa. Instead, you will create your own tasty menus and decide if you want a couple of snacks each day or not. Your goal is to shed pounds without sacrificing your overall health. The recommended dietary intakes and suggestions of the USDA Food Guide Pyramid are useful guides. They have been formed from the culmination of thousands of studies and expert contributions from not just the United States, but around the world. Nutritional scientists and obesity experts have played a role in helping the government extract important information from field studies and converting it to recommendations.

Whenever you make changes in your diet, large or small, your body kicks up an automatic fuss, because your body strives for homeostasis—a feature of our physiology that has helped our species survive. The key to getting through the initial backlash phase is to make sure that your expectations are realistic and your mind is focused on the mission ahead. You have to believe in yourself and erase your history of past diet failures. Those other diets were for short-term weight loss, but this is the diet that will set you up for the rest of your life. Visualize a slimmer, healthier, happier you right from the very beginning, and hold on to that image, especially when you seem to be stuck at a plateau. If you've created a positive aura about what you're trying to do, it will help block out all of the potential negative forces that try to steer you off the course of success.

I don't have a magical food plan that will burn away the fat in a matter of weeks and guarantee a certain amount of weight loss. What I will offer you, however, is a chance to control your own diet, make choices that appeal to your taste, and still lose weight. It's what I like to call the "flex diet," because you're in charge of what you eat for each meal and how much. The guidelines that follow will remind you of the amount of calories that correspond to meeting your desired weight loss goal.

The first thing that you must do is a bit of record keeping. Before you decide where you're going, you must know your starting point. Choose a day to begin monitoring your consumption and record everything—except for the air you breathe—that enters your mouth. Even half a glass of milk must be recorded. This consumption log should be kept over a seven-day period, and it must be as accurate as possible. Honesty is the only way that this consumption log will help or the food plan be effective. Resist the urge to jump-start your diet by curbing your consumption during the week you're keeping the log. Instead, it's important that you eat, drink, and snack as you normally do. Besides recording quantity, detailing the times is important. One day's consumption log might look something like this:

7:30–9:00
English muffin with butter
1 scrambled egg
2 pieces of bacon
1 glass of orange juice

11:30–11:35
2 chocolate-chip cookies

12:30–1:15
chicken breast sandwich with mayo, tomato, cheese
small garden salad
1 bag of barbecued potato chips
1 can of Coke

2:30–2:45
1 can of Coke

3:15–3:35
1 bag of M&M's

5:30–5:40
1 can of Coke
1 glazed doughnut

7:30–8:30
mixed vegetables
fettuccini Alfredo with bits of bacon and cream sauce
2 white rolls
1.5 glasses of wine
2 scoops of chocolate ice cream

10:30
3 Oreo cookies
½ glass of milk

Once you've logged a week's worth of consumption, it's time to do all of the math. Using charts available at the end of this chapter, find the food consumed or what's most similar on the chart. Match as closely as possible the servings that you ate of the food, then calculate the amount of calories in each food. For example, the breakfast just listed would measure as follows:

1 buttered English muffin	169
1 scrambled egg	100
2 pieces of bacon	201
1 glass of orange juice	106
Total breakfast calories	**576**

For caloric and nutrient descriptions of many types of foods and preparations, see "Composition of Common Foods and Beverages" in the appendix (page 201). However, it's impossible to list every food and the variety of ways it can be prepared. This exercise is just to get a rough estimate of your consumption, so don't be afraid to find the closest food sample on the chart and estimate.

Once you have calculated the daily caloric consumption, you might have a log that reads something like this:

MON.	TUES.	WED.	THURS.	FRI.	SAT.	SUN.	TOTAL
2,350	2,600	3,200	2,100	2,875	2,455	2,800	18,380

$$\frac{18,380}{7} = 2,626 \text{ cal/day}$$

Our goal is to take one pound off per week through calorie-intake reduction. One pound equals 3,500 calories. So if you're going to lose a pound through diet changes alone, you must average a calorie reduction of 500 per day. Thus, if you are a person who consumes on average 2,626 calories per day, you would have to adjust your diet so that you now consume 2,626 − 500 = 2,126 calories. If you're able to follow the plan for a month, that would mean four pounds shed simply through reducing your portions and cutting back on all the fattening snacks. Notice I didn't say eliminating, just cutting back. The backbone of the flex diet is that you don't starve or deprive yourself of your favorite foods. It means that you will now make smart choices and consume calorie-rich food in moderation.

Admittedly, this 500-calorie-a-day reduction will be tough for some. If, however, you remember the overall goal of a 3,500-calorie reduction per week, then you might decide to take advantage of the flexibility of the program and eat 400 fewer calories one day, then 600 the next to make up for it. The reason I suggest a daily reduction of 500 is that it's typically easier to spread the calorie reduction over several days instead of one. So our thirty-day plan would look something like this:

	MON.	TUES.	WED.	THURS.	FRI.	SAT.	SUN.	TOTAL
Week 1	-300	-500	-400	-600	-600	-500	-600	-3,500
Week 2	-500	-500	-200	-700	-600	-700	-300	-3,500
Week 3	-400	-400	-500	-600	-700	-500	-400	-3,500

	MON.	TUES.	WED.	THURS.	FRI.	SAT.	SUN.	TOTAL
Week 4	-500	-500	-400	-500	-400	-600	-600	-3,500
Total							14,000 calories = 4 pounds	

One caveat must be mentioned for those who are already consuming fewer than 2,000 calories per day. Reducing caloric intake by 500 means falling below the 1,500-calorie mark, which is probably the lowest many people can handle within healthful parameters. For example, if your consumption log states that you consume only 1,800 calories per day, then reducing this by 500 leaves 1,300 calories, which might be too low to meet minimum energy requirements. Remember that even during your efforts to lose weight, the body still must carry out basic functions and you must be able to participate in activities. If you don't have a sufficient amount of energy, two things can ensue that become counterproductive to your efforts. Your metabolism—another important way to expend energy—will automatically slow and reduce the amount of calories burned. Second, your energy supply will be so drastically reduced, you won't have the strength to participate in the physical activities that are another important part of our program (discussed in chapter 10).

Following are a series of menus for breakfast, lunch, and dinner. They're divided into 300, 400, 500, and 600 calories. You can use them as a guide for what you select to eat. You also have the flexibility to choose from the different menus. For example, let's say that you should be consuming 2,000 calories per day to lose one pound per week. You might choose a 300-calorie breakfast, 500-calorie lunch, 600-calorie dinner, and two 300-calorie snacks to give you a total of 2,000 calories. Feel free to use the tables at the end of this chapter to find your favorite foods to create your own menus. You can switch and swap as much as you like as long as you don't exceed your daily calorie limit. If, however, you do exceed it one day, just eliminate a snack the next day and make up for it. It's that simple, and it's all under your control.

BREAKFAST

300-CALORIE OPTIONS

1 English muffin, toasted
2 tsp. peanut butter
¾ cup plain low-fat yogurt
¾ cup blackberries

1 cup bran cereal
1 cup 1% milk
1 medium banana
½ cup orange juice

2 4-inch pancakes
1 tbsp. sugar-free syrup
1 cup skim milk

1½ cups puffed wheat
1 cup skim milk
1 cup cantaloupe

1 minibagel
2 tsp. jelly
1 tbsp. cream cheese
1 cup skim milk

400-CALORIE OPTIONS

1 English muffin, toasted
2 tbsp. peanut butter
¾ cup plain low-fat yogurt
¾ cup blackberries

1 cup Bran cereal
1 cup 1% milk
1 large banana
1 cup orange juice

3 4-inch pancakes
1 tbsp. sugar-free syrup
1¼ cups strawberries
1 cup skim milk

1½ cups puffed wheat
1¼ cups skim milk
1 cup raspberries
1 small nectarine

1 minibagel
2 tsp. jelly
1 tbsp. cream cheese
1½ cups skim milk
2 tbsp. raisins

500-CALORIE OPTIONS

2 slices whole-wheat bread, toasted
1 egg, scrambled
1 tsp. butter
1 slice American cheese
1 cup 1% or skim milk
1 medium banana

½ cup oatmeal
2 cups raspberries
1 English muffin, toasted
1 tbsp. reduced-fat margarine
¼ cup low-fat cottage cheese
1 cup 1% or skim milk

1 cup whole-grain cereal
1¼ cups strawberries
1 cup 1% or skim milk
1 egg omelet
1 minibagel, whole-wheat, toasted
1 tbsp. reduced-fat margarine

(continues on following page)

(*500-Calorie Options*, *continued*)

2 low-fat waffles
1 tbsp. syrup
1 tbsp. reduced-fat margarine
1 cup orange juice
1 cup low-fat yogurt
½ large grapefruit

½ bagel, whole-wheat
1 tbsp. cream cheese
2 slices tomato
1 cup cranberry juice
1 cup 1% or skim milk
2 medium plums

600-CALORIE OPTIONS

2 slices whole-wheat bread, toasted
2 eggs, scrambled
1 tsp. butter
1 slice American cheese
1 cup 1% or skim milk
1 large banana

½ cup oatmeal
2 cups raspberries
1 English muffin, toasted
2 tbsp. reduced-fat margarine
½ cup low-fat cottage cheese
1 cup 1% or skim milk

1 cup whole-grain cereal
1¼ cups strawberries
1 cup 1% or skim milk
1 egg omelet
1 oz. shredded American cheese
1 minibagel, whole-wheat, toasted
1 tbsp. reduced-fat margarine

3 low-fat waffles
1 tbsp. syrup
2 tbsp. reduced-fat margarine
1 cup orange juice
1 cup low-fat yogurt
½ large grapefruit

½ bagel, whole-wheat
1 tbsp. cream cheese
2 oz. smoked salmon
2 slices tomato
1 cup cranberry juice
1 cup 1% or skim milk
2 medium plums

LUNCH

300-CALORIE OPTIONS

1 6-inch pita
3 oz. canned tuna
1 tbsp. reduced-fat mayonnaise

2 slices whole-wheat toast
2 oz. lean roast beef
1 tbsp. mustard
lettuce and tomato

1 cup tomato soup
24 oyster crackers
1 green apple
½ cup fat-free frozen yogurt

1 cup split pea soup
2 cups mixed salad greens
2 tbsp. reduced-fat salad dressing
½ cup skim milk

(continues on following page)

(300-Calorie Options, continued)

2 cups mixed greens
2 tbsp. vinegar and oil
2 oz. feta cheese

400-CALORIE OPTIONS

1 6-inch pita
4 oz. canned tuna
2 tbsp. reduced-fat mayonnaise
lettuce and tomato

2 slices whole-wheat toast
2 oz. lean roast beef
1 slice provolone
1 tbsp. mustard
lettuce and tomato

1 cup tomato soup
24 oyster crackers
1 green apple
12 almonds
½ cup fat-free frozen yogurt

1½ cups split pea soup
2 cups mixed salad greens
3 tbsp. reduced-fat salad dressing
½ cup skim milk

2 cups mixed salad greens
2 tbsp. vinegar and oil
2 oz. feta cheese
1 whole-grain roll, small
1 tsp. reduced-fat margarine

500-CALORIE OPTIONS

2 slices whole-wheat bread
3 oz. lean roast beef
2 slices tomato
1 tsp. mayonnaise
½ cup fresh fruit salad

1 large flour tortilla
3 oz. grilled chicken breast
1 tsp. mayonnaise
½ cup mixed salad greens
1 tbsp. oil and vinegar
1 orange

½ bagel, whole-grain
2 oz. fresh roasted turkey, skinless
1 tsp. mustard
2 cups mixed salad greens
1 tbsp. Russian dressing

4 large sesame breadsticks
2 cups mixed salad greens
3 oz. canned tuna
2 tsp. mayonnaise
1 large pear

1 slice pizza with vegetables
1 cup mixed salad greens
1 tbsp. Italian dressing

600-CALORIE OPTIONS

2 slices whole-wheat bread
3 oz. lean roast beef
2 slices tomato
1 tsp. mayonnaise
½ cup fresh fruit salad

(continues on following page)

(600-Calorie Options, *continued)*

1 large flour tortilla
3 oz. grilled chicken breast
1 tsp. mayonnaise
½ cup mixed salad greens
1 tbsp. oil and vinegar
1 orange

½ bagel, whole-grain
2 oz. fresh roasted turkey, skinless
1 tsp. mustard
2 cups mixed salad greens
1 tbsp. Russian dressing

4 large sesame breadsticks
2 cups mixed salad greens
3 oz. canned tuna
2 tsp. mayonnaise
1 large pear

1 slice pizza with vegetables
1 cup mixed salad greens
1 tbsp. Italian dressing

DINNER

300-CALORIE OPTIONS

1 6-inch taco shell
2 oz. flank steak
1 tsp. canola oil
¼ cup salsa
½ oz. shredded cheddar cheese

8 oz. tofu
1 cup cooked broccoli
2 tsp. olive oil

⅔ cup couscous
2 oz. shrimp, grilled
1 cup cooked carrots
1 tsp. olive oil

2 oz. ground sirloin
1 cup rigatoni
1 cup cooked tomatoes

2 cups chow mein
⅓ cup white rice
1 cup cooked water chestnuts

400-CALORIE OPTIONS

1 6-inch taco shell
2 oz. flank steak
2 tsp. canola oil
¼ cup salsa
1 oz. shredded cheddar cheese

8 oz. tofu
1½ cups cooked broccoli
2 tsp. olive oil
⅓ cup brown rice

⅔ cup couscous
3 oz. shrimp, grilled
1½ cups cooked carrots
2 tsp. olive oil

3 oz. ground sirloin
1 cup rigatoni
1 tsp. olive oil
1 cup cooked tomatoes

2 cups chow mein
⅓ cup white rice
3 oz. skinless, boneless chicken
   breast
1 cup cooked water chestnuts

500-CALORIE OPTIONS

1 cup pasta
4 oz. baked skinless, boneless
    chicken breast
2 cups grilled vegetables
2 tsp. olive oil

1 cup white rice
1 cup lentils
2 cups cooked mixed vegetables
1 tsp. butter
1 peach

1 6-oz. potato, white
4 oz. sirloin steak
2 cups broccoli, cooked
1 tsp. canola oil

4 oz. baked salmon
⅔ cup brown rice
1 cup green beans, cooked
1 cup Romaine lettuce
2 tbsp. oil and vinegar

4 oz. skinless, boneless chicken
    breast
1 oz. low-fat shredded Mexican
    cheese
½ cup salsa
2 6-inch flour tortillas
⅓ cup Spanish rice

600-CALORIE OPTIONS

1 cup pasta
5 oz. baked skinless, boneless
    chicken breast
2 cups grilled vegetables
2 tsp. olive oil
2 small tangerines

1 cup white rice
1 cup lentils
2 cups cooked mixed vegetables
1 tsp. butter
1 peach
3 gingersnaps

1 6-oz. potato, white
5 oz. sirloin steak
2 cups broccoli, cooked
2 tsp. canola oil

5 oz. baked salmon
⅔ cup brown rice
1 cup green beans, cooked
2 cups Romaine lettuce
2 tbsp. oil and vinegar

6 oz. skinless, boneless chicken
    breast
1 oz. low-fat shredded Mexican
    cheese
1 cup salsa
2 6-inch flour tortillas
⅓ cup Spanish rice

SNACK MENUS

100 CALORIES	200 CALORIES
⅓ cup plain low-fat yogurt dip and 2 cups raw vegetables	6 slices melba toast topped with ¼ cup ricotta cheese
2 graham cracker squares and 2 tsp. low-sugar jelly	1 small pita, toasted, topped with ⅓ cup hummus
15 grapes and ½ cup skim milk	2 cups honeydew melon and ½ cup plain low-fat yogurt
½ cup plain low-fat yogurt	½ cup sorbet and 2 vanilla wafers
2 tbsp. raisins and 10 peanuts	1 medium doughnut (1½ oz.)
2 gingersnaps and ½ oz. cheddar cheese	1 granola bar and 15 cherries
2 chocolate-chip cookies (e.g. Chips Ahoy)	1/12 angel food cake (unfrosted), topped with 1¼ cup strawberries and 2 tbsp. whipped topping and ½ cup skim milk
½ small package licorice (e.g. Twizzlers)	¼ cup Grape-Nuts mixed with 1 tbsp. raisins and 1 cup skim milk
4 animal crackers and 1 small orange	1½ oz. pretzels and 5 almonds
2 rice cakes topped with 1 tsp. peanut butter	1 cup skim milk plus 1 tbsp. chocolate syrup and 1 small tangerine
1 cup unsweetened applesauce	1 oz. potato chips dipped in ¼ cup salsa
1 medium banana, frozen	1 brownie (2 inches), unfrosted, and ¾ cup skim milk
8 halves dried apricots and ½ cup skim milk	1 small mango and 10 cashews
½ cup sugar-free chocolate pudding (made with skim milk) topped with 2 tbsp. whipped topping	¾ oz. baked tortilla chips topped with 1 oz. of melted cheddar cheese and ¼ cup salsa
6 saltine-type crackers topped with 2 tsp. low-sugar jelly	1 green apple, sliced with 1 tbsp. peanut butter and 1 cup skim milk

Refer to the appendix, "Composition of Common Foods and Beverages" (page 201), for an extensive list of food items that you can substitute for the sample menus above, keeping in mind that you want to replace menus items with foods that have the same caloric values. Also, "How to Read a Food Label" (see appendix, page 224) will provide you with an explanation of how to read a food label so that you can calculate your caloric intake accurately.

YOUR GOAL in using these menus should be to plan your meals in advance, one day at a time. Remaining conscious of what you're eating will ensure that you stay within your allotted calorie-intake goals and will also help you develop an instinct for how much food your body needs to lose weight and maintain your desired weight. The process of losing weight gradually and in a healthful manner is useful in itself, as you will have developed new habits that can last a lifetime by the time you reach your goal.

As you utilize these menus, pay attention to your levels of energy and hunger and adjust your caloric intake to your satisfaction. You should not skip meals, but you may find that you need to power through the day with a substantial breakfast and lunch in exchange for a light meal at dinnertime. You may also find that you do not need two snacks in between meals to maintain your energy level, in which case you can eat larger and more varied meals.

Naturally, you will not always be in control of every meal. Make an effort, even when dining out, to eat portions equivalent to the suggestions above. Most restaurants serve larger portions of food than we actually need. When dining out, you might quickly assess the portions on your plate and decide in advance how much you should eat. Vigilance and consistency will result in success.

PART FIVE

GET A GRIP ON YOUR WORKOUT

CHAPTER 10

SWEAT THE SMALL STUFF

The Benefits of Physical Activity and Exercise

All parts of the body which have function, if used in moderation and exercised in labours in which each is accustomed, become thereby healthy, well developed, and age more slowly, but if unused, they become liable to disease, defective growth, and age quickly.

HIPPOCRATES

EXERCISE AND PHYSICAL ACTIVITY FIGHT FAT

Declining physical activity is, perhaps, the primary cause of a global increase in obesity and overweight, with Americans leading the statistical charge.

The Surgeon General's 1996 Report on Physical Activity has documented just how little Americans are participating in exercise or vigorous activity. Only 15 percent of U.S. adults engage regularly—three times a week for at least twenty minutes—in vigorous physical activity during their leisure time. Approximately 22 percent of all adults engage regularly—five times a week for at least thirty minutes—in sustained physical activity of any intensity during leisure time. The most disturbing statistic: One in every four adults reports no physical activity at all during their leisure time. The report also goes on to detail important disparities in physical activity; most notably, men are more active than women, whites are more active than African Americans and Hispanics, and the more wealth one possesses, the more likely he or she is to engage in physical activity.

According to a panel of scientists convened by the Centers for Disease Control and the American College of Sports Medicine, enough evidence exists to demonstrate the health benefits of regular, moderate-intensity physical activity. Exercise promotes cardiorespiratory fitness, thus aiding in the prevention of heart attack, lung disease, and circulatory system problems. Exercise also helps the body absorb glucose from the blood, reducing the risk for diabetes. Quantities of fat that store dangerous and detrimental elements can be burned off with routine physical activity. Exercise also reduces cholesterol levels and lowers blood pressure by making the blood vessels more elastic and better able to expand according to the pressure the blood exerts against its walls. Moreover, exercise triggers the release of the body's natural endorphins, thereby mitigating discomfort from chronic pain and acting as an antidepressant. Other noteworthy side effects of sweating it out include healthier and more efficient digestion, clearer skin, and improved metabolism.

The role that physical activity and exercise can play in fighting overweight cannot be overstated. Several studies have shown that those who lose weight through dietary changes alone are more likely to regain the weight, because they eventually return to their predieting eating habits and without increased activity, have no way of burning the excess calories. Those who have been most successful at losing weight and keeping it off for longer periods of time have typically included some regimen of exercise or increased their level of physical activity. Add an exercise component to your dietary changes, and you'll increase your chances of losing weight. If one method doesn't work as well as you like, you'll at least have the other to pick up the slack.

The effect of exercise on body fat has been a subject of study by scientists for decades and confirms what most of us know, experientially, to be true. The Centers for Disease Control and the American College of Sports Medicine recommend that every U.S. adult should accumulate thirty minutes or more of moderate-intensity physical activity on most, preferably all, days of the week. Moderate-intensity physical activity is defined as enough to expend approximately 200 calories per day. A few ways to burn this number of calories would be to walk two miles briskly, play golf and carry your clubs for forty minutes, or spend fifty minutes painting your home.

While the ideal way to obtain the benefits of exercise is through a continuous thirty-minute period of exertion, experts have found that breaking up the activity throughout the day can still yield benefits. You can meet the physical activity recommendation through short bouts of exertion, whether it's walking up the stairs instead of taking the elevator, walking instead of driving short distances, or pedaling a stationary bicycle while watching television. If you prefer the lower-intensity activities, simply do them more often for longer periods of time.

Exercise generally affects body composition and weight favorably by promoting fat loss while preserving or increasing lean muscle mass. The rate of weight loss is positively related to the frequency and duration of the physical activity session, as well as to the duration of the physical activity program. The rate of weight loss through just physical activity adjustments can be slow, but adding dietary changes such as reducing calorie loads can help boost the speed with which you'll lose the weight and your chances of keeping it off for a longer period of time.

Ignoring the important contribution that exercise plays in reducing and maintaining one's weight may be the most common mistake dieters make. Many of my patients have enthusiastically related stories about the amazing amount of weight they lost on the latest fad diet. Sadly, most of these hopeful dieters typically regained the weight they lost—and sometimes additional pounds—when they couldn't stick to an eating regimen that was unnatural to them. Most people who lose weight rapidly on crash diets do not engage in an exercise or physical activity program, because the weight initially comes off so easily that they don't feel the need. However, a panel of experts convened by the National Institutes of Health made it very clear in their consensus report on obesity that food restriction alone was not adequate in the majority of cases to trigger permanent weight loss. A review of the literature made it abundantly clear that those who participate in a program that combines food changes as well as increased activity lose the most weight and are able to keep it off the longest.

EXERCISE VS. PHYSICAL ACTIVITY

For most of the book I've been mentioning exercise and physical activity, and you're probably wondering why am I making a point to mention both when in essence they are the same thing. In fact, there are important differences. Understanding these differences can better help you classify which of the two you most often participate in. You will also be able to make a better-informed decision as you craft a program that's more tailored to your specific needs and schedule. Both can affect your level of energy expenditure, but the amount of time you put into each one to reach the same energy output can be drastically different.

> **PHYSICAL ACTIVITY:** Any bodily movement produced by skeletal muscles that results in energy expenditure.

> **EXERCISE:** A subset of physical activity defined as "planned, structured, and repetitive bodily movement done to improve or maintain one or more components of physical fitness."

PHYSICAL ACTIVITY AND WEIGHT LOSS

While exercising on a climbing machine, riding a stationary bicycle, or jogging on a treadmill are often the fastest ways to increase your energy expenditure and burn those calories, they aren't the only ways to meet your goals. You can burn calories and shed pounds in the course of your everyday life by increasing your participation in physical activities. Activities like taking a walk in the neighborhood, planting flowers in the garden, or washing the car can be important and effective methods of burning fat and bringing your weight under control. See "Caloric Expenditure During Various Activities" in the appendix (page 226) for a detailed chart of activities and their corresponding caloric requirements. It takes more time using these physical activities to burn the same number of calories as you would with exercise, but it can be done, and for those who don't want to run on a treadmill, engaging in a variety of physical tasks is a viable alternative.

EXERCISE AND WEIGHT LOSS

When most people think of exercise, they usually imagine hot gyms filled with scantily clad, lean bodies dripping with sweat that look as if they are being filmed for a sportswear commercial.

Understandably, this stereotypical perception of exercise—an exhausting and competitive grind in a large, multilevel gym that plays loud music and punishes those who skip a week of working out—is either intimidating or a turnoff. I've interviewed many people who prefer not to exercise at all if it entails going to a gym and enduring painful workouts with other people who are so well conditioned that it's an embarrassment to be in the same room. Certainly, joining a gym and/or attending classes can be intimidating at first, as many new experiences are. If the convenience of belonging to a gym enables you to take control of your exercise schedule, however, don't let fear or awkwardness stand in the way. Ignore everyone else. You are doing this for yourself, not for an audience—real or imagined. Many people I have counseled have been reluctant to join a gym, but once they have done so, they find the support of other members, the regularity of their routine, and the camaraderie that can develop in exercise classes a great boost.

Exercise, undeniably, is about attitude—not a competitive one, but a determination to submit your body to a physical stress that in the long run will improve your physical stature, overall health, and mental energy. You have to believe in the exercise and what it can deliver to you. A large part of taking control is making well-thought-out decisions about the path that will lead to your goals. Take charge of how you expend energy and try to enjoy losing the weight and tuning up your cardiovascular and respiratory systems in the process.

If you've always had an aversion to exercise, you might consider thinking about why you haven't done it in the past and whether its potential benefits are strong enough to convince you to try. Preconceived negative notions only hinder you and do little to open your mind to the great possibilities. Exercise is often an individual journey, because you begin to learn about your body, spirit, and sense of determination. Even in the midst of others, you're really alone as you challenge your muscles to lift more, your heart to beat faster, and your will to power you through the toughest part of the workout. It's the relationship with your body that you develop during exercise that helps you gain a greater respect for your body's amazing machinery. The more you work for physical improvement, the more conscious you'll be about feeding your body healthy foods and keeping fit. Feeling good makes you want to feel even better, and this begins an exciting cycle of working out, losing weight, eating well, and staying your course.

AEROBIC VS. ANAEROBIC EXERCISE

A lot of research has been conducted on the benefits of aerobic exercise versus those of anaerobic exercise, but the differences between the two haven't been made abundantly clear. In simple language, aerobic exercise is any extended activity that causes your heart, lungs, and vascular system to work harder than when at rest, using the large muscle groups (hips, legs, chest, and back) at a regular, even pace. Aerobic exercises use a large amount of oxygen, increase your metabolism, and burn fat (not blood glucose) for fuel. The major health benefit beyond burning fat is the cardiorespiratory fitness that results from a prolonged regimen of aerobic exercises. Examples of aerobic exercises include brisk walking, jogging, swimming, bicycle riding, aerobic dancing, Rollerblading, or skiing.

To get the most benefits from aerobic activity, you should be exercising at a level strenuous enough to raise your heart rate to your target zone. This zone is calculated as taking 50–75 percent of your maximum heart rate, which itself is defined as 220 minus your age. This is how a forty-year-old person would calculate the exercise target heart rate:

> 220 − 40 = 180 (maximum heart rate)
> 50% of 180 = 90
> 75% of 180 = 135
> target heart rate zone = 90–135 beats per minute

It's easy to check if you're reaching this target zone. In the middle of your exercise, place your index and second fingers on the underside of your wrist to feel the pulse of your radial artery. An easy way to find the pulse: First place your fingers in the middle of the muscle bulge at the base of your thumb. Then slide the fingers directly back toward your wrist. You'll begin to feel the pulsation of your heart within one to two inches of the starting point in your hand, at the level of the wrist. Count the number of pulse beats for fifteen seconds, then multiply this number by four to get the number of beats per minute. You can also get this recording by feeling the pulse beats in the carotid arteries on the sides of your neck. The best place to find your pulse is just below the angle of the jaw. Apply a little pressure into your neck until you feel the pulse.

This target heart zone is a good guide to whether you're exercising too hard or not hard enough. Adjust the intensity of your exercise until your heart rate falls within the calculated target zone range. You should exercise within your target zone, because exceeding it can over-stress the capacity of your heart and lungs and result in an inadequate amount of blood being pumped by the heart, thus making your work-out less effective and even detrimental to your health. For patients who are predisposed to heart disease, this is especially important, as exces-sive work placed on the heart can lead to oxygen deprivation in the heart muscle—ischemia—and cause a heart attack.

Aerobic exercise does very little to tone the muscles, if anything at all. Typical aerobic workouts require your muscles to perform hun-dreds of repeated contractions, but little resistance is placed on them. Resistance through loading—such as lifting weights—is the ideal way to stimulate muscle development and tone. I've heard people suggest that for aerobic exercises to be effective at burning fat, they must be conducted at a low intensity. While exercising within your target heart rate yields the most efficient results, fat loss can be achieved regardless of the intensity of the exercise.

Anaerobic exercise is performed without the use of breathed oxy-gen; instead, other fuel sources such as glucose are required to carry out the exercise. Anaerobic exercises use muscles at high intensity and a high rate of work for a short period of time. Anaerobic exercises help increase muscle strength and require short bursts of energy. The work of these exercises occurs so fast and with such a demand, it exceeds the potential use of the oxygen that we breathe. Examples of anaerobic exercises include sprinting and weight lifting, essentially any exercise that requires a rapid burst of energy.

Anaerobic exercises, unlike aerobic exercises, can't be performed for long periods of time because the muscles run out of fuel and quickly reach exhaustion. These exercises are also limited in duration by the accumulation of lactic acid, a by-product of the breakdown of glucose. Before you can repeat another anaerobic exercise at maximal levels, the body must burn up the lactic acid during a recovery period. The ideal length of time and intensity of your anaerobic exercise depends on factors that are unpredictable and difficult to calculate. The amount of lactic acid that accumulates is virtually impossible to measure. You have to listen to your body. If your muscles cramp or you become extremely fatigued, stop. Pushing yourself after you are fatigued could spell disaster for your aching muscles and other soft tissues that are vulnerable to tears and sprains.

Anaerobic exercises aren't as efficient as aerobic exercises at burning calories and thus reducing body fat. They do, however, increase the strength and size of the skeletal muscles. This can be important in reducing fat, because while it is not possible to convert fat to muscle, the larger the muscle mass, the greater the body's overall energy requirement. A pound of muscle uses 35–50 calories more per day than a pound of fat. Even while at rest, skeletal muscles require a certain amount of energy for simple metabolic needs. Anaerobic exercises can also be good for improving cardiovascular fitness and reducing risk factors such as total cholesterol and blood pressure.

TAKE YOUR TIME

Start slow. This advice applies to anyone who has not been active over the last year. Rushing into physical activities and exercises can actually do more harm than good. It's important not to overdo it as you begin your exercise program. Muscles that have not been stressed for a long time, or never at all, are prone to injury. You should begin by closely monitoring your heart rate and adjusting your effort so that your heart rate is close to the lower endpoint of your target zone for thirty minutes. As your body, including your heart, becomes more efficient, your increased endurance will allow you to up the intensity of your workout to the upper endpoint of the target zone for longer periods of time.

EXERCISE AND DIABETES

When I was a second-year medical student, I received a call from home. "Ian, Grandma has diabetes," my mother said. Those words ricocheted in my head until they finally settled and left me with an overwhelming feeling of numbness and hopelessness. I was the only one with any medical or scientific background in the family, but I was in the middle of a tough semester, hundreds of miles from home. I wanted to call and reassure her, but I didn't know enough about the disease and its treatments to sound convincing. I immediately dove into my textbooks and gave myself a crash course about a disease that afflicts as many as sixteen million Americans.

After getting a handle on the causes and methods of diagnosis, I carefully read the treatment options available, ranging from the most aggressive to the conservative. Beyond medications, about which I knew she would be apprehensive, I discovered that weight loss and exercise played an important role in not only reducing the levels of blood sugars, but also potentially eliminating the need for powerful medications. The several studies that had been cited noted a significant drop in the level of circulating glucose and a reduction in how much sugar-lowering medications were required to keep the sugar under control. What I liked most about this connection between exercise and diabetes management was that the physical activity requirement wasn't beyond the capability of even a seventy-year-old grandmother. There are many activities in which people of various ages and levels of fitness can participate, such as walking, a few times a week to reap the impressive benefits of weight reduction and increased metabolic activity.

When I went home after the semester, I was fully versed in the treatment of diabetes and the role exercise could play in controlling it. When I explained the disease to my forlorn grandmother, I assured her that there was hope that she could reduce the level of diabetes medications she was taking and eat a more normal diet. The one catch, I explained, was that she was going to have to start exercising or finding some way to increase her level of physical activity. She agreed reluctantly to visit the gym with my twin brother and me, so we got her a little workout suit and she began her first workout regimen by walking on the treadmill for ten minutes.

The change in attitude and spirit that my grandmother underwent was nothing short of amazing. No longer did we have to cajole her to go to the gym with us; she would actually call us to see if we would pick her up on our way! After a few weeks she had made several friends at the gym, and her workouts increased to twenty minutes on the treadmill, followed by short rides on the stationary bicycle. She called us one afternoon with the greatest sense of accomplishment after visiting the doctor. He was amazed at how much her blood sugar level had dropped and wanted to know if she had been doing anything different. She, of course, proudly told him about her workout regimen and how much better it made her feel. The proof wasn't only in her more positive demeanor about tackling the diabetes, it was also apparent in the laboratory results, which after a couple of months of exercising were so much improved that he cut back on her diabetes medications.

My grandmother was just one of millions of Americans with type II diabetes who could benefit significantly from a regular routine of vigorous exercise or physical activity. In fact, doctors have been so encouraged about the benefits of exercise in helping diabetics that they've begun recommending it immediately to patients who are mild to moderate diabetics, realizing the exercise can have the synergistic effect of lowering blood sugar levels.

Medical literature is full of the positive response that diabetics experience with exercise. Several studies involving college alumni, female registered nurses, and male physicians have demonstrated that physical activity protects against the development of diabetes. In a study of male university alumni, researchers found that physical activity was inversely related to the incidence of diabetes. The greater the level of physical activity, the lower the risk for developing diabetes. Each 500 calories of additional leisure-time physical activity per week was associated with a 6 percent decrease in diabetes risk. In a study of female registered nurses age thirty-four to fifty-nine years, women who engaged in vigorous physical activity at least once a week had a 16 percent lower adjusted relative risk of reporting diabetes during eight years of follow-up, compared to women who reported no vigorous physical activity.

Researchers believe exercise helps prevent and treat diabetes by increasing the body's sensitivity to insulin, the important hormone released by the pancreas that allows the cells in the body to absorb the glucose from the blood. The more effective insulin is at carrying out its tasks, the more glucose is absorbed from the blood and used as energy. In fact, exercise can be such an important adjunct to medications that the American Diabetes Association has recommended that an appropriate exercise program be added to diet or drug therapy to improve blood glucose control and reduce certain cardiovascular risk factors among diabetics. Doctors believe the exercise works not only to help make the body more sensitive to insulin—and thus allow greater absorption of glucose from the blood—but also to reduce the amount of stored fat, which has been shown to predispose overweight people to diabetes.

CHAPTER 11

CHOOSE YOUR WEAPON

Customizing Your Exercise Routine

N ow it's time to customize an activity program that will get you on the road to weight loss and improved health. There are, however, a few housecleaning chores that you should follow up on before getting started. If you've been inactive for a year or more, it's important to see your doctor for a thorough physical exam regardless of your age and current or previous level of fitness. Changing your dietary habits as well as increasing your physical workload can provide an enormous amount of physical and psychological benefits, but this combination of changes can also put your body through a large amount of stress. Most healthy people can adequately adapt to this physical stress without any problems, but certain underlying conditions can be worsened by the demands of increased physical activity. If you have an irregular heartbeat, respiratory problems such as asthma or chronic obstructive pulmonary disease, or metabolic disturbance in which your body's chemistries are abnormal, you could be putting yourself in grave danger by exercising without medical clearance. You might look and feel good, but it can't be overstated that there are many silent medical conditions that are detectable only through laboratory work or a physician's careful examination. The demands of increased physical activity are so great that they can bring conditions that are brewing quietly to a loud boil.

Even if you already know that you have a medical condition and it's been well controlled under treatment, you still need to check in with your doctor to make sure it's all right to begin a program and confirm the acceptable level of intensity. In addition, regardless of your general health, I recommend a full physical exam before you begin a regular and possibly strenuous exercise program. Even professional athletes have suffered from undiagnosed medical problems, sometimes with fatal consequences.

Once your doctor gives you the okay, it's time to take a little inventory, just as you did before starting the dietary changes. It helps to get a rough idea of how much energy you're currently expending. This will help you set realistic activity goals and clarify a starting point from which you can build a lifelong activity plan. Pick any day of the week, and the minute you roll out of bed make sure you record as much as possible about your physical activities. It's not necessary to record every waking minute, but activities that take a lot of time such as typing for three hours or standing for a significant period need to be recorded. It's especially important to include all activities that burn energy, such as washing windows for thirty minutes or walking home from work. Keep as accurate a time count as possible, as the activity and amount of time you spend in that activity are crucial in calculating your daily energy expenditure through physical activity. The journal's entry, of course, ends as you get into bed and resumes the next morning when you wake.

This type of record keeping isn't fun, but it's crucial to be diligent and honest about your activity log. It doesn't help if out of guilt you suddenly take up activities that you've never participated in before just so your log doesn't show how sedentary a life you otherwise lead. You're the only one looking at this log, and you're the one customizing the exercise plan, so you'll only be cheating yourself if you suddenly decide to change your typical activity roster. Keep this journal for seven days. At the end of the week you'll total the amount of calories burned, then calculate a daily average. There are, of course, some days that you might spend more time being sedentary, whether it's watching a couple of hours of television or sitting through a class. There will be other days that you will be busier running errands, walking to the store, or playing a game of tennis. In order to construct a program that works best for your schedule and includes the activities that you enjoy, keep the times as specific as possible.

A sample entry might look something like this:

Monday, July 22, 2001

> 7:00 A.M. Awake
>
> 7:30 A.M. Shower/dress
>
> 8:00 A.M. Breakfast
>
> 8:25 A.M. Drive car to work
>
> 9:00 A.M. Arrive at work and begin day
>
> 9–12:00 P.M. Working-related activities, nothing strenuous
>
> 12–1:00 P.M. Lunch and a 1-mile walk on company grounds
>
> 1–4:30 P.M. Finish work
>
> 4:30–5:15 P.M. Drive home
>
> 5:45–6:30 P.M. Clean the house, do laundry
>
> 7–8:00 P.M. Walk ½ mile to gym/participate in 30-minute aerobics class
>
> 8:30–9:00 P.M. Walk home
>
> 9:15–10:00 P.M. Warm up and eat last night's leftovers
>
> 10:30–11:30 P.M. Surf the Internet and watch television
>
> 11:45 P.M. Off to bed

At the end of the week, highlight all of the physical activities and the amount of time you spent performing them. To get a rough estimate of the calories you burned for the day through physical activities, check "Caloric Expenditure During Various Activities" (see appendix, page 226). Record the amount of calories you use each day in your dieter's log. A one-week log might look like this:

MON.	TUES.	WED.	THURS.	FRI.	SAT.	SUN.
1,400	1,900	2,300	1,750	2,400	1,200	1,100

Week's Total: 11,050

Daily Average: 11,050 cal./7 days = 1,579 cal. per day

Now that you've calculated the number of calories expended per day, you can begin to devise an exercise or physical activity regimen that works best for you. For the first week of your new exercise program, the goal is to expend an average of 250 calories per day, giving a week's total of 1,750 expended calories. This is equal to half a pound.

That may sound like a lot of work for little pay, but don't wave this off as insignificant. You'll also be losing a pound through your dietary changes. Depending on your schedule, it might be easier to divide up the activities over three, five, or all seven days. Some will find it easier to participate in regularly scheduled activities that involve others, such as a weekly game of basketball or a day of gardening at the local park. Group participation can be an important motivator for many, because others come to expect your contribution and you feel obligated not only to yourself but also to others and the advancement of a team goal. Whether it's helping to plant fifty new bushes in the park or playing pickup basketball with your friends every Thursday night, your focus mustn't be on doing the activity simply to meet the day's energy expenditure requirement. Instead, your participation should be driven by a desire to accomplish something in which you've made a physical and emotional investment.

The mental strategy of taking control of your physical activities can be a make-or-break situation for those who are either increasing their participation after a long time of being sedentary or simply have little desire to increase the demands on their body. How you visualize and perceive a physical activity program can be just as important as carrying out the tasks. A positive outlook means viewing the activity not as a chore, but as an undertaking whose results you share a genuine interest in bringing to fruition. People who enjoy the work that they do don't sit at their desks watching the clock every half hour to see how close they are to the next break or end of the day. People who truly enjoy their work must often force themselves to leave the office for lunch or be cajoled by their colleagues to leave a project and complete it tomorrow. When your physical activity begins to feel like an inconvenience, then the smallest of deterrents or excuses can throw you off course.

A key aspect of the take-control diet is that the physical activity or exercise program that you choose is completely under your direction. An activity prescription that will burn off a set amount of calories per week, but that you find uninteresting or unable to do because of scheduling conflicts, is of little help to you. Instead, you must decide how you plan to burn those excess calories in the spirit of making long-term life changes. This book should simply guide you in the right direction, providing you with the necessary information to make the most informed decision possible.

Your activity program is as important as the dietary changes you make. It's crucial that you pick activities that you like and will continue for at least a year, or even potentially for a lifetime. However, this doesn't mean that you can't switch activities. If gardening is one of your important activities, you might want to change to another during the winter months when the ground is frozen. The essence of the exercise program is flexibility. The choices are yours, and you should be comfortable with them and feel excited to begin your program.

Our first week is more of a warm-up week to get our bodies adjusted to the idea of increased daily activity. We'll start by expending 1,750 calories, which is equivalent to half a pound. This means that the goal for a five-day week is 350 calories per day. This doesn't mean, however, that you can't spread this out over all seven days, which would equal 250 calories per day. For some people, seven days might be too much and they would prefer to finish the physical activity regimen over a shorter period of time and rest for a couple of days. Your physical activity plan has the same guiding principle as the diet—flexibility. You can choose to expend more energy one day and less the next, use three weekdays and the two weekend days, or divide the 1,750 between two major activities. (This approach should only be taken by those in reasonably good shape.)

MON.	TUES.	WED.	THURS.	FRI.	SAT.	SUN.	TOTAL
350	350	350		350	350		1,750

To burn this amount of energy, take a look at "Caloric Expenditure During Various Activities" in the appendix (page 226) and choose the activity/activities of your preference to be carried out vigorously for at least thirty minutes. You might choose to perform the activity for a longer period of time, which will give you a great energy output, or you might choose more than one activity. Whatever combination you choose is fine, as long as you meet the 350-calorie expenditure goal for the day. Here's a sample of activities that would meet this goal for a 150-pound woman:

Bowling	53 minutes
Kickboxing	35 minutes
Car washing	73 minutes
Frisbee toss	51 minutes
Walking (brisk)	65 minutes
Washing windows	76 minutes
Racquetball	29 minutes

These activities and their energy burn are only examples, but remember, whatever activity you choose and how long you choose to perform it can vary any way you want as long as you're enjoying it and are meeting your goal. You might decide to do more than one thing, so your activities for one day could look something like this:

Activity-Minded Person

Monday
Washing windows—30 min.
(138 cal.)

Gardening—digging/hedging—20 min.
(172 cal.)

Food Shopping—10 min.
(42 cal.)

Day's Total Calorie Burn: 352 cal.

Sports-Minded Person

Monday
Frisbee toss—20 min.
(136 cal.)

Running (11.5 min. miles)—17 min.
(156 cal.)

Rowing machine (moderate pace)—10 min.
(81 cal.)

Day's Total Calorie Burn: 373 cal.

Now it's important to return to the physical activity log that you kept the first week. The task before you is to classify the activities according to their energy demand—low, moderate, or high. One of the important goals of your activity program is to replace the low-energy activities with those requiring a higher input of energy. If you have moderate-energy activities, try to replace those with higher-demanding activities. If you enjoy your activities and they already require a moderate energy demand, try to simply increase the amount of time you spend performing those activities. Following are some physical activity samples and their corresponding energy requirements. For purposes of reference, we'll use a 170-pound man. Energy expenditures will vary according to physical activity as well as the gender and weight of the participant. The heavier you are, the greater the energy expenditure, and for some activities, men expend more energy than women for the same amount and intensity of activity. (Refer to "Caloric Expenditure During Various Activities" in the appendix, page 226, for a full list.)

Basketball	11.4 cal./min.
Bowling	7.5
Carpet sweeping	3.7
Cleaning	4.5
Food shopping	4.8
Gardening (hedging)	5.9
Roller-skating	9.0
Typing	2.1
Walking (asphalt road)	6.2

Source: Katch and McArdle, *Introduction to Nutrition, Exercise, and Health*, 4th ed. Baltimore, MD: Lippincott Williams & Wilkens, 1993.

If your activity log lists food shopping and walking as two important energy-burning activities, then you might want to consider increasing the length of the walk or replacing it with a more vigorous exercise such as roller-skating. (It would be difficult to change the amount of time you spend food shopping unless you decide to do your neighbor's shopping also.) If you don't want to roller-skate, but wouldn't mind bowling once a week, then add this to your physical activity roster. Take control of what works best for you, and feel free to switch or swap and increase or decrease activities.

Now that you've completed the first week and you've worked out most of the kinks, it's time to rev the engine a little more. There are several ways you can accomplish this, either by increasing the intensity of your activities, doing the activities for a longer period of time, or adding a new activity to the plan. If you're going to add a new activity and most of your plan has been low-intensity, then try a moderate-intensity activity, one with more vigor. I think it's good to add an aerobic activity (jogging, swimming, cycling, dancing) because it will help increase your cardiovascular fitness and burn fat the fastest. Aerobic exercises, depending on the intensity, can burn calories quickly, efficiently, and enjoyably. If we keep to our philosophy of gradually turning up the program each week, the exercise goal of the second week is to lose approximately ¾ pound through exercise. This would mean increasing your calorie burn to 2,625 over the entire week. If you've chosen the five-day plan, you will need to burn 525 calories per day. The seven-day plan requires that you burn 375 per day. Once again, refer to the tables in the appendix to decide which activities work best for you while trying to accomplish this goal.

Our third and fourth weeks will be where we start to settle into a comfortable stride. You've had two weeks to get adjusted to the dietary program and activity plan, and now it's time to find the pace that you can continue comfortably for an indefinite period of time. Your goal is to take control for the rest of your life, not to just make it to the next event. The goal of the third and fourth weeks will be to lose a pound each week through activities. This means burning 3,500 calories a week, an amount that equals 700 each day if spread over five days or 500 each day if spread over a seven-day period. This is a big commitment, but if you're determined to take control of feeling and looking better, then you'll be pleased with the results. To summarize the thirty-day activity plan for a five-day week:

	MON.	WED.	FRI.	SAT.	SUN.	TOTAL
Week 1	350	350	350	350	350	1,750
Week 2	525	525	525	525	525	2,625
Week 3	700	700	700	700	700	3,500
Week 4	700	700	700	700	700	3,500
Total						11,375

A total of 11,375 calories for the month means 3 1/4 pounds lost through exercise alone. Don't forget that you've also been sticking to the flex diet. That means 1 pound per week, for a total of 4 pounds for the entire month. If you take the total program combined, you've lost 7 1/4 pounds in just one month! This is only the beginning. As you adjust to your healthier style of eating and exercising, all this will become second nature and you'll be able to make these choices without first having to check to make sure you're eating fewer calories and exercising more.

CALCULATING CALORIC BURN

As you attempt to calculate the number of calories you're burning through exercise or physical activity, be aware that it's virtually impossible to calculate your precise caloric burn. When using devices that calculate the calories you've burned, such as monitors on stationary bicycles or treadmills, remember that they aren't exact. The number the machine reports is simply an estimate, with an error factor of 5 to 25 percent. However, the estimates provided on most exercise equipment or in the appendix of this book will more than serve your purposes.

One of the purposes of exercising is to get your heart, muscles, and lungs in shape. Over a period of time, consistent activity will begin to tune up these different systems, and your body will become more efficient at using oxygen and consuming energy. As you get in better shape, your body will require exercises of greater intensity or longer duration to continue to improve. Look at this in a positive light; it means the activity plan is working.

A WORD ABOUT WHEN TO EXERCISE

There is no unanimous answer among fitness experts about the best time to exercise. Certainly, working out in the morning can give your metabolism a boost as you carry on with the day's activities. People often talk about the "exercise high" they get after working out in the morning that can last through most of the day. And exercising an hour or so after a meal can be beneficial to immediately counteract those consumed calories, but it's not critical that you exercise after each meal. Some people prefer to exercise at night—not a bad idea as long as you don't do it too close to bedtime. Exercising and then going to sleep shortly thereafter blunts the metabolism boost you might have otherwise enjoyed had you not gone into a restful slumber (which automatically slows your metabolism).

PART SIX

CALL THE SHOTS
IN YOUR OWN GAME

CHAPTER 12

A BRAND-NEW LIFE

Hopefully by the time you've reached this point of the book you are motivated and excited about developing new behavior patterns to take off extra pounds, maintain your new weight, and enjoy a robust and improved life. Those who are most successful at losing weight are concerned not only about being able to fit into a particular size of clothing, but about improving their overall heath and fitness. There is no prescription that any doctor can write or drug that any company can manufacture that will guarantee your health. And that is a good thing. You are in control of your health.

For many people, taking control won't be a major endeavor, it will be a matter of fine-tuning some areas that are slightly out of key. For others, getting on the road to a brand-new life will mean major changes, a long commitment, and refusing to allow plateaus and setbacks to dampen their determination. This book begins with a chapter on the mental edge, because without a positive mind-set your body's natural resistance to change will overcome your will to make changes. Only you can summon the strength to address those personal factors that have influenced your eating behaviors and physical activity schedule. Diet books might provide the plans, but those plans are only as good as your execution of them.

Taking control is more than just a diet program. It's a decision to reinvigorate your life and get behind the steering wheel. If our lives weren't limited, there would be less urgency to eat the right foods and participate in physical activity to keep the body fine-tuned. The truth of the matter is that we have a limited time on this earth and need not waste it fighting diseases that are preventable through good lifestyle choices and a character-building dose of discipline.

The next few sections of this book address common temptations and pitfalls you may encounter. A general mantra for success in overcoming temptation is "Play on your own team." Understand that cheating is self-sabotage. Permitting a momentary lapse in which you sneak a high-calorie snack is depriving yourself of success—not indulging yourself in a treat. Caving in to a craving is like scoring a point for the other team. Conversely, every day, taking one day at a time, that you adhere to your diet and exercise plan, you are scoring your way to a lasting personal victory.

SURVIVING THE HOLIDAY TEMPTATION

One of America's sacred cultural customs is celebrating the holidays in grand style. Cheer and grand feasts are two mainstays of celebrations. The biggest challenge for most people is enjoying the festivities and all the delicious foods without overindulging and packing on those holiday pounds. The first step in prevention, of course, begins with the mind. Believing that it's inevitable to put on those extra holiday pounds is a setup for failure. Your attitude before sitting down to a big meal or entering a company holiday party full of rich foods and heavy desserts must be one of vigilance. Just because the food is there doesn't mean it has to be eaten.

Ironically, with all the talk about holiday pounds, most people don't gain as much as they think they do. The findings of a recent study in the *New England Journal of Medicine* contradict the popular belief that most people gain between five and ten pounds between Thanksgiving and New Year's Day. Researchers found that most Americans probably gain only about a pound during the winter holiday season. The concern is not over that one pound, but over what happens if the extra weight defeats your resolve and triggers a relapse into old patterns of behavior or accumulates through the years and contributes to overweight later in life.

There are several ways you can stop yourself from overindulging during these food extravaganzas. The simple act of consciously realizing what a calorie splurge will do to all the hard work that you've put into maintaining control over your energy consumption and output will serve as a major deterrent from participating in costly behaviors. Following are a few tips that can help you get through the holidays without packing on the pounds.

PLAN AHEAD   Often, the success of weight loss programs, especially during the vulnerable times of holiday, comes down to good planning. It's better to have a course of action for the different situations you might encounter, rather than be caught off guard. For example, think ahead of time about what you'll do when you're offered those high-calorie foods. Play out the anticipated scenes in your mind, reacting to the situation with self-control and poise. It might even be better to have the scenario written down, a concrete reminder of what you'll expect and your prepared response, both verbally and physically.

Company parties are often rife with temptation because you have little control over the foods that are served, and they are typically loaded with fats and high-calorie items that do not provide fiber, nutrition, or the ability to sate your appetite. If you know that you'll be attending a party, actually sit down and try to map out your day's calorie plans, making sure you won't exceed the preset daily calorie limit that you've already been following. Remember, the advantage of the flex diet is that it allows you to exchange menu items with different calorie counts. Make use of this if the company party is going to be near a mealtime—lunch or dinner. Instead of eating one of those meals and eating at the party, simply let the party food serve as a substitution for that meal. Let's say, for example, the party is at eight o'clock and you're on a 2,000-calorie plan. If you choose to eat a 300-calorie breakfast and 400-calorie lunch and skip the snacks, you'll save a whopping 1,300 calories for the party. This would typically be a bigger dinner than you are accustomed to eating, so when you get home from the party, change into something comfortable and take a quick walk. Or, if you own a stationary bicycle, take a thirty-minute ride to burn off some of those calories. This could also help kick-start your metabolism right before going to bed, when your metabolism typically settles at its slowest pace through the night.

YOU BE THE COOK Another way to avoid the excess holiday poundage is to actually take control of what you're eating by cooking some of the food yourself. If you're hosting the party, then you can easily prepare special dishes that are low in calories but still tasty. If you're a guest at someone else's home, you might make a tactful suggestion to bring a couple of dishes for the party, and this is your opportunity to reduce the fat and increase the vegetables.

VEG FOR A DAY If you're in a situation where all of the foods offered to you are full of those fattening calories, veg out—that's right, just eat vegetables. Typically, hosts will prepare at least a couple of vegetable dishes to accommodate the vegetarians in the group. There are also fruit dishes, such as a fruit platter or fruit salad. These aren't always the lowest in fat, but they may be your healthiest choices. Fruits and vegetables contain fiber and have a low energy density that will fill you up yet not pack in the calories.

AVOID ALCOHOL Alcohol and parties seem to go hand in hand, but that doesn't have to be. Don't forget, every gram of alcohol has an extremely high energy density of 7, making it second only to fat, which has an energy density of 9. Many people don't realize that a good portion of their extra calories comes from the amount of alcohol they consume. Drinking alcohol not only sends your calorie intake into orbit, it can also weaken your resolve. Moreover, alcohol slows down the metabolism so that your body burns calories at a rate below whatever is normal for you. Try substituting sparkling water with a twist of lime or cider for wine or champagne—it will taste different, but the carbonation is festive and having a glass in your hand can be satisfying by itself. One way to ensure that you don't drink is by volunteering to be the designated driver, fully aware that drinks and driving don't mix.

BECOME A PICKY EATER It's completely unrealistic to expect to pass through a holiday season without eating some of your favorite foods. Let's be honest: Delicious foods are prepared for these big occasions, and it's difficult for even the most determined of us to resist the urge to eat some of what we love. Remember, the spirit of the flex diet is not to eliminate completely, but to reduce the consumption of your favorite high-calorie foods. So if you're going to be offered a variety of foods, rather than sample everything, save your calories for those foods you most enjoy. When you do get a chance to dig in, however, make sure you do it in moderation.

EAT SLOWLY   One of the mistakes we make when presented with what seems like a limitless amount of food is to eat everything quickly, perhaps in response to the sheer abundance before us or because we've skipped a meal in anticipation of the feast. If you eat slowly, you'll continuously send signals of fullness to the brain, keeping in mind that it takes about twenty minutes for enough signals to be sent to dissipate your hunger. The slower you eat, the greater the chance that you will not be tempted with second helpings.

KEEP SOMETHING IN THE TANK   It's important to make sure you don't go to a party hungry or save your appetite for a big meal at the end of the day. You could cut down on how much you eat at the party by eating a smaller meal before the party. Buffet tables are a disaster waiting to happen, so avoid them unless you are able to choose selectively and there are healthy options. Having a little fuel in the tank before you survey the long banquet table might help you keep your portions small and prevent you from making return trips.

KEEP YOUR JOURNAL   You might have put your journal away since you've been well along on your plan, but the holidays are a great time to dust it off and put it to use. It will keep you honest with yourself, especially since memories can become selective (when we do something we know we shouldn't do). The holiday season seems to be the optimal time to develop eating amnesia, so the journal can serve as a method of making sure you stick to your food plan.

KEEP EXERCISING   This is not a good time to start sliding on your exercise program; in fact, if there's a time that's most important to keep up with your program, it's during a holiday. It's completely understandable that you might eat a few extra calories over the course of a holiday. Counteract the additional calories with extra exercises or physical activities. If you increase the energy input, you need to increase the energy output to keep your weight stable. I often advise people who are preparing to go to an event that will be offering lots of fattening foods to simply match the added calories with added exercises. The more you eat, the more you exercise and the greater the likelihood that you'll keep those unwanted party pounds off your waistline.

SURVIVING VACATIONS

Like holidays, vacations are a prime opportunity for people to forget about all their hard work and return to their old habits of eating as much as they want of whatever they want. Society has formed an "anything goes" attitude about vacations: it's all right to cheat, because you're supposed to be getting away from the everyday stresses of your life. Unfortunately, this attitude and subsequent behavior is only a setup for disaster. People not only eat and drink an enormous amount while on vacation, they tend to spend most of their time sedentary, forgetting the exercise or activity schedule that they have been following at home. It is important that when you vacation you don't take a vacation from your diet and exercise plan.

Vacations should be enjoyed. When you work hard and endure life's numerous daily grinds, it's important to put your mind and body at ease, to catch up on your rest and relaxation. This, however, doesn't mean that you still can't eat healthfully and stay active. You simply have to make the necessary preparations that allow you to at least adhere to most of your daily routine. Follow some of these tips for a healthier vacation.

COOK YOUR OWN MEALS   If you're going on a short vacation to a place where you can store food in a refrigerator and heat it up in a microwave oven or stove, cook some of your meals at home and bring them along with you. This is an excellent way to control the portions and calories of the food you eat. It will help you avoid one of the biggest weight traps, fattening restaurant meals and calorie-rich fast-food fare.

ALTERNATE YOUR MEALS   Eating new and interesting cuisine is a major attraction when vacationing in a foreign land. It's unrealistic and not even desirable to ignore the aromas of a tasty dish and opt for safer, familiar food whose calorie count you know. It's difficult to keep track of your calories with foods that you haven't eaten before or haven't helped prepare. So in the spirit of vacation, spend one day eating moderate portions of the indigenous foods. Next day stick to the foods you're more familiar with and can keep better track of. This approach doesn't deprive you of foreign culinary delights, but it will help keep you from packing in calories and regretting it when you return home. With a little effort you can be healthy on vacation and have fun. Your enjoyment will, in fact, be enhanced as you stick to your plan in a new environment rather than feeling victimized by it.

SIGHT-SEEING IS KEY   Depending on where you go, make sight-seeing one of your daily activities. This allows you to kill two birds with one walk—enjoy the sights of your traveling destination and keep down your caloric intake at the same time. You can get an extra benefit by choosing a walk that courses through more hilly terrain, requiring you to walk up and down, stressing your muscles and pushing your endurance. If you're not in the middle of viewing a sight, make that walk between the two points brisk enough to increase your heart rate.

CHOOSE YOUR LODGING CAREFULLY   Where you stay on vacation can be the greatest determinant of whether you'll get an adequate amount of exercise or physical activity. Once again, thinking ahead is key. Choose a place that has amenities such as a swimming pool, gym, tennis court, or any type of sporting facility. It's much easier to motivate yourself to exercise when it's just a matter of taking the elevator downstairs to the gym or heading outside for a swim. Make sure you pack the trunks and pair of sneaks and you'll be in business.

TUNE UP BEFORE VACATION   If your vacation is planned well enough in advance, consider using the week before you leave to get ahead. Decrease your caloric intake and accelerate your exercise or physical activity enough to burn up extra calories and put yourself ahead of schedule. This will serve almost like an insurance policy in case you're not able to keep the food calories down and work off enough fat.

GETTING AROUND THE COMMON PITFALLS

I've attempted to be completely honest with you about the amount of effort it takes to lose weight and keep it off. I could sell you on a program that guarantees thirty pounds in sixty days with no need to exercise, but a few days on the diet and you would soon learn the absurdity of such promises. I hope that by this point you're convinced that losing weight isn't easy, but it's certainly something you can accomplish if you're willing to take control and live your life for yourself. Many great military strategists have said in their own way that one of the keys to battle is knowing as much as possible about the enemy. Along the way to dieting success, you will certainly encounter some common pitfalls. If you know what they are, you will be prepared to navigate around them.

Stuck in the Same Gear

Weight plateaus are every dieter's nightmare. You've been losing weight steadily for a few weeks and all of a sudden the scale keeps registering the same number. You're still watching what you eat and sticking to your food plan, as well as participating in vigorous activities—yet the weight appears to be stuck. Peaks and valleys and steady plateaus are a simple reality of weight loss programs, but it's important to realize that most of it has nothing to do with your efforts or dedication to the program. Understanding how the body is programmed to lose weight might help shed light on why you reach plateaus and help you break through them.

As I've mentioned earlier, the first pounds that come off are the easiest, while the rest are more difficult, coming off gradually. As you begin to lose weight, your muscles strengthen, and your body adjusts to a healthier and more physically fit you, the program that was working earlier won't be as effective. A plateau is often your body saying, "I'm too good now, you're gonna have to come at me with a bigger challenge."

Once we start losing weight, those billions of cells begin to shrink. The more they shrink, the more they feel as though they're being starved. This sense of starvation is not what we want, because it triggers the body's natural tendency to prevent excessive weight loss. The body's response to this fat cell shrinkage and perceived starvation is to slow down metabolism, thus decreasing the rate at which we burn energy. The more starved the body feels, the more it wants you to believe that you're hungry and need to eat more. If you obey the instinct to eat, the pounds creep back.

When you reach one of these plateaus and feel like scrapping your diet altogether, it's important to shift your focus not on the weight you're trying to lose, but on the health benefits you expect from sticking to the program. Taking control is not just a program to get you into a smaller bathing suit next summer. It's about making a lifelong commitment to yourself and your quality of life. Even if you are not losing weight at the moment, eating less saturated fat and participating in more aerobic activities will continue to be beneficial in guarding against the onset of such health problems as cardiovascular disease, high blood pressure, cancer, and type II diabetes. The desire to feel better and live longer will reinforce your willpower so that you can continue your program with vigor. Plateaus occur when the body needs to readjust to a new diet and the physiological changes brought on by weight loss. Eventually, the now shrunken fat cells will adjust to their new size and cease sending false starvation messages to your brain. This may take a few weeks, but if you stay the course, you'll plow right through the plateau and begin losing weight again.

Setbacks

I've never met anyone successful at losing weight who didn't experience times along the way where they either consumed an inordinate amount of calories or simply stopped exercising for a week or two—sometimes for unavoidable reasons. These setbacks are normal and to be expected. It's like a game of basketball. Watch two good teams play and follow the score changes that occur in one single game. Team A is up by ten points, then team B makes a comeback and cuts the lead down to two points. Team A makes another run and pushes its lead back up to eight points before team B has an amazing three minutes of play and scores twelve points in a row, now taking the lead by four points. Team A finally wins the barn burner of a game by a score of 103–98, but it was a hard-fought game that at several times along the way could've gone to either team.

Dieting is often a battle between losing the weight and gaining a small portion back, having a great three weeks of following the food and activity plan, then having a week where your body just doesn't want to follow the program anymore. Right from the very beginning, you must accept that these minor setbacks will occur throughout your life, but it's the positive mental edge that will allow you once again to take control and get back on course. Don't let these minor interruptions in your winning schedule become major disruptions in the game of life.

Many people enter programs expecting their path to be smooth riding, no rocks or bumps along the way. When they do meet a minor hindrance, they're caught so off guard that they don't have the willpower or confidence to grab the reins and get the horse trotting again. You must develop a plan before you begin your program that maps out how you're going to handle these inevitable setbacks. Develop what I call an emergency plan that can be put into action the minute you realize you're on a downward slide. Your emergency plan might consist of a meal plan that reduces your caloric intake by 700 calories a day instead of the 500-calorie reduction that has been your routine. You can also include an exercise augmentation, increasing the length of your exercise or physical activities by 25 percent. So if you walk for thirty minutes a day, you'll now be walking 37½ minutes. If you've had only a mild setback, this emergency plan shouldn't have to be enacted for more than a week or two, enough to get you back in the saddle and heading in the right direction.

Humor and optimism, not frustration and anger, must constitute your outlook. It's all right to be disappointed in yourself for slipping, but do not let your discouragement slide into self-punishment. Too often, people get so angry at themselves that they throw up their arms in resignation and totally dismiss the weight loss program and, even more sadly, dismiss themselves as a complete failure. If you can laugh at your errors and weaknesses, then you're more likely to call yourself a funny name, shake your head, and shrug off the 3,500-calorie day simply as a temporary lapse. Pencils have erasers on one end and a point on the other because everyone makes mistakes. Keeping your mind pegged to this reality and occupying positive space will increase your chances of success when encountering these small pockets of failure.

Despite your best efforts to be realistic in setting your weight goals, you still might have stretched your expectations. Let's say you find yourself in a common predicament. You've gone through all the careful steps of keeping a consumption and activity log, calculating your calories, and choosing a menu that allows you to reduce your caloric intake by 500 calories per day. You've followed this plan diligently, yet the scale isn't registering the number of pounds you expected to lose. If this happens over four weeks, then you should reconsider and reassess your goals.

You can first try adjusting your food and activity plan, challenging yourself to eat fewer calories and participate in more vigorous activities. You might then want to adjust your weight loss schedule, where instead of losing a pound or more a week, you lose a pound every two weeks for a certain period of time, then go back to a pound a week. We must accept the fact that our bodies are different and how they respond to the same program will vary. The thirty-day program I've outlined is simply a guide, not a hard and fast rule of what will happen if you follow it. Some people will lose more weight than anticipated, while others will lose less.

USE REWARDS

What good is being good if you don't get some type of reward? The biggest reward of this program is that you'll feel your life is in your control. You will lose weight, look better, and feel great. It's important to reward your hard-won efforts through mechanisms that will serve as positive reinforcement.

We teach children by reinforcing their good behavior or task accomplishment. When they learn how to spell their names or feed themselves, we applaud their efforts and often reward them with some type of gift to let them know that their accomplishment is recognized and appreciated. Positive reinforcement is effective, instilling in children the principle that hard work can lead to success and that success deserves recognition. As adults, our professional success is often recognized, whether by way of an "Employee of the Month" award or some honorable mention in the company newsletter. But when it comes to losing weight and improving your health, only you know how difficult it was to stick it out, and you should do the rewarding, whether it's a new pair of shoes, a new golf club, or a trip you've been wanting to take.

Some people find it helpful to set up a reward system just as they do a food or activity schedule. For two pounds you might buy yourself a shirt, for eight pounds a new purse, and for twelve pounds a nice bracelet. These rewards can go all the way up till you reach your final weight goal, where you award yourself the biggest prize. Reaching this weight goal, however, is half the battle. Now you must be able to keep the weight off. Many of the gimmick diets leave you at this point, allowing you to figure out on your own how to maintain your weight, but the essence of the take-control diet is that the knowledge you have gained about food, weight, and your body will carry you through the rest of your life. The techniques and principles that you learned during the first week of your diet are the same ones you should follow the thirtieth week.

Rewarding yourself for weight maintenance may also be an effective way of keeping off the excess weight. Some people enter arrangements with their companions or friends that reward them for keeping the weight off for three months, six months, twelve months, and so on. The goal is to reach a point physically and psychologically where you no longer need a reward to motivate your efforts or confirm that you've been successful. The goal is to make eating right and taking part in a sufficient amount of physical activity second nature. It becomes such a normal part of your routine that you wouldn't pay it any more attention than you do your morning rituals.

LOOKING TO THE FUTURE

My hope is that as you incorporate the customized flex diet into your life and start participating in more physical activity, you will cease feeling as though you are on a diet. Rather, with patience and discipline, you can experience a brand-new way of living. Keeping a journal of the foods you eat and your daily activities is a good way to get your mind trained to these new lifestyle choices, but once you have adopted new habits you will not need to scribble down every bite of a sandwich or sip of soda. Journals are a simple exercise in retraining your mind to think more closely about what you're eating and doing, with the aim that after a while you can put them away. The behavior modifications and lifestyle choices that you've made will become part of who you are. Losing weight is only part of this program, but the bigger aim is building a lifelong self-confidence. You will have the mental edge that allows you to find and then tap into those hidden spaces of your soul, special reserves of energy, and determination that will give you an inner strength to improve your appearance and your health. The first day you begin to take control is the first day of your new life. Step boldly and with determination in this direction of ultimate health and freedom, and your success will fuel greater confidence in yourself—confidence that will, in turn, manifest in all areas of your life. You can do this.

APPENDIX

BODY MASS INDEX (BMI)

Height	18	19	20	21	22	23	24	25	26	27	28	29	30	31	32	33	34	35	36	37	38	39	40
										Body Weight (pounds)													
4'10"	86	91	96	100	105	110	115	119	124	129	134	138	143	148	153	158	162	167	172	177	181	186	191
4'11"	89	94	99	104	109	114	119	124	128	133	138	143	148	153	158	163	168	173	178	183	188	193	198
5'0"	92	97	102	107	112	118	123	128	133	138	143	148	153	158	163	168	174	179	184	189	194	199	204
5'1"	95	100	106	111	116	122	127	132	137	143	148	153	158	164	169	174	180	185	190	195	201	206	211
5'2"	98	104	109	115	120	126	131	136	142	147	153	158	164	169	175	180	186	191	196	202	207	213	218
5'3"	102	107	113	118	124	130	135	141	146	152	158	163	169	175	180	186	191	197	203	208	214	220	225
5'4"	105	110	116	122	128	134	140	145	151	157	163	169	174	180	186	192	197	204	209	215	221	227	232
5'5"	108	114	120	126	132	138	144	150	156	162	168	174	180	186	192	198	204	210	216	222	228	234	240
5'6"	112	118	124	130	136	142	148	155	161	167	173	179	186	192	198	204	210	216	223	229	235	241	247
5'7"	115	121	127	134	140	146	153	159	166	172	178	185	191	198	204	211	217	223	230	236	242	249	255
5'8"	118	125	131	138	144	151	158	165	171	177	184	190	197	203	210	216	223	230	236	243	249	256	262
5'9"	122	128	135	142	149	155	162	169	176	182	189	196	203	209	216	223	230	236	243	250	257	263	270
5'10"	126	132	139	146	153	160	167	174	181	188	195	202	209	216	222	229	236	243	250	257	264	271	278
5'11"	129	136	143	150	157	165	172	179	186	193	200	208	215	222	229	236	243	250	257	265	272	279	286
6'0"	132	140	147	154	162	169	177	184	191	199	206	213	221	228	235	242	250	258	265	272	279	287	294
6'1"	136	144	151	159	166	174	182	189	197	204	212	219	227	235	242	250	257	265	272	280	288	295	302
6'2"	141	148	155	163	171	179	186	194	202	210	218	225	233	241	249	256	264	272	280	287	295	303	311
6'3"	144	152	160	168	176	184	192	200	208	216	224	232	240	248	256	264	272	279	287	295	303	311	319
6'4"	148	156	164	172	180	189	197	205	213	221	230	238	246	254	263	271	279	287	295	304	312	320	328
6'5"	151	160	168	176	185	193	202	210	218	227	235	244	252	261	269	277	286	294	303	311	319	328	336
6'6"	155	164	172	181	190	198	207	216	224	233	241	250	259	267	276	284	293	302	310	319	328	336	345

UNDERWEIGHT	HEALTHY WEIGHT	OVERWEIGHT	OBESE
(<18.5)	(18.5–24.9)	(25–29.9)	(≥30)

Find your height along the left-hand column and look across the row until you find the number that is closest to your weight. The number at the top of that column identifies your BMI.

Source: From A. Must, G. E. Dallal, and W. H. Dietz, "Reference Data for Obesity: 85th and 95th Percentiles of Body Mass Index (wt/ht²) and Triceps Skinfold Thickness." *American Journal of Clinical Nutrition* 53 (1991): 839–846. Adapted with permission by the *American Journal of Clinical Nutrition*, © *American Journal of Clinical Nutrition*, American Society for Clinical Nutrition.

THE ENERGY DENSITY SPECTRUM FOR SELECTED FOODS

CATEGORY 1: VERY LOW-ENERGY-DENSE FOODS (0 TO 0.6 CALORIES PER GRAM)

Water	0.0
Lettuce	0.1
Tomato	0.2
Strawberry	0.2
Broccoli (cooked)	0.3
Salsa	0.3
Grapefruit	0.3
Vegetarian vegetable soup	0.3
Cantaloupe	0.4
Milk, skim	0.4
Winter squash	0.4
Applesauce	0.4
Carrots	0.4
Chicken, rice, and vegetable soup	0.5
Italian dressing, fat-free	0.5
Orange	0.5
Yogurt, fat-free with aspartame	0.5
Vegetarian chili	0.5
Yogurt, fat-free, plain	0.6
Blueberries	0.6
Apples	0.6

CATEGORY 2: LOW-ENERGY-DENSE FOODS (0.6 TO 1.5 CALORIES PER GRAM)

Tofu	0.6
Milk, whole	0.6
Oatmeal, prepared with water	0.6

Mayonnaise, fat-free	0.6
Cottage cheese, fat-free	0.7
Grapes	0.7
Black beans	0.8
Green peas	0.8
Corn on the cob (boiled, drained)	0.9
Orange roughy (broiled)	0.9
Banana	0.9
Sour cream, fat-free	0.9
Yogurt, 99% fat-free	1.0
Pudding, vanilla, prepared with 2% milk	1.0
Cottage cheese, regular (full-fat)	1.0
Cheerios with 1% milk	1.1
Tuna, canned in water	1.1
Crispix with 1% milk	1.1
Potato, baked with skin	1.1
Veal chop, braised	1.2
Yogurt, fat-free, vanilla	1.2
Frozen yogurt, fruit varieties	1.3
Rice, white, long-grain, cooked	1.3
Ham, extra lean, 5 percent fat	1.3
Turkey breast, roasted, no skin	1.4
Ranch dressing, fat-free	1.4
Spaghetti, cooked	1.5

CATEGORY 3: MEDIUM-ENERGY-DENSE FOODS (1.5 TO 4.0 CALORIES PER GRAM)

Egg, hard-boiled	1.6
Chicken breast, roasted, no skin	1.7
Hummus	1.7

(Category 3: Medium-Energy-Dense Foods, continued)

Ham, 11% fat	1.8
Sirloin steak, lean, broiled	1.9
Pork chop, center loin, broiled	2.0
Pumpkin pie	2.1
Margarine, low-calorie	2.1
Apricots, dried	2.4
Bread, whole-wheat	2.5
Grape jelly	2.5
English muffin	2.6
Angel food cake	2.6
Mozzarella cheese, part-skim	2.6
Ranch dressing, reduced-fat	2.7
Potato chips, fat-free	2.7
Italian bread, white	2.7
Bagel, plain	2.8
Raisins	3.0
Potatoes, French-fried	3.2
Mayonnaise, light	3.3
Doughnut, jelly-filled	3.4
Cream cheese, full-fat	3.5
Fruit chewy cookies	3.6
Italian dressing, full-fat	3.6
Butter, light	3.6
Chocolate cake with frosting	3.7
Licorice, cherry	3.7
Swiss cheese	3.8
Hard pretzels	3.8
Popcorn, air-popped, plain	3.8

Rice cakes, plain	3.9
Tortilla chips, baked	3.9

CATEGORY 4: HIGH-ENERGY-DENSE FOODS (4.0 TO 9.0 CALORIES PER GRAM)

Graham crackers	4.2
Chocolate-chip cookies, homemade	4.6
Tortilla chips	4.6
Creme-filled chocolate sandwich cookies	4.9
M&M's, plain	4.9
Bacon	5.0
Potato chips	5.4
Milk chocolate bar	5.4
Peanuts, roasted	5.9
Ranch dressing, full-fat	5.9
Peanut butter, creamy	5.9
Pecans, dry roasted	6.6
Mayonnaise, regular, full-fat	7.1
Butter	7.2
Margarine, stick	7.2
Oil, vegetable	8.8

Source: Barbara Rolls, Ph.D., and Robert Barnett, *Volumetrics Weight-Control Plan* (New York: Harper-Collins, 2000).

FIBER CONTENT OF FOODS

To consume more fiber, eat more whole fruits and vegetables, whole grains, and beans. Nuts are also rich in fiber, but they are energy dense, so eat them in small amounts. Use the following list to guide your food choices. It is adapted from research conducted by the Tufts University School of Medicine in Boston and published in the *Tufts Health & Nutrition Letter.*

FRUITS*	GRAMS OF FIBER
Apple (with skin)	4
Banana	3
Blueberries, ½ cup	2
Cantaloupe, 1 cup diced	1
Dates, ⅛ cup dry, chopped	2
Grapefruit, ½	2
Grapes, 1 cup	2
Nectarine (with skin)	2
Orange	3
Peach (with skin)	2
Pear (with skin)	4
Plum (with skin)	1
Prunes (dried), 10	2
Raisins, ⅛ cup	1
Raspberries, ½ cup	4
Strawberries, ½ cup	2
Watermelon, 1 cup diced	1

VEGETABLES†	GRAMS OF FIBER
Broccoli, ½ cup cooked, chopped	2
Broccoli, ½ cup chopped	1

*All values are for 1 medium-size fruit unless otherwise indicated.

†All values are for raw, uncooked vegetables unless otherwise indicated.

Brussels sprouts, ½ cup cooked	3
Carrot, 1 medium	2
Carrots, ½ cup cooked	3
Cauliflower, ½ cup cooked	2
Celery, 1 stalk	1
Corn, ½ cup cooked	2
Cucumber, ½ cup sliced	0.5
French fries, 1 small (2.5 ounces) serving	2
Green beans, ½ cup cooked (frozen)	2
Iceberg lettuce, 1 cup shredded	1
Peas, ½ cup cooked (frozen)	4
Peppers, ½ cup chopped	1
Potato, baked, with skin	5
Potato, baked, without skin	2
Potato, ½ cup mashed	2
Romaine lettuce, 1 cup shredded	1
Spinach, ½ cup chopped	1
Spinach, ½ cup cooked (frozen)	3
Sweet potato, baked with skin	3
Tomato, 1 medium	1

GRAINS, LEGUMES* (BEANS, CHICKPEAS, LENTILS, LIMA BEANS), AND NUTS

GRAINS, LEGUMES* (BEANS, CHICKPEAS, LENTILS, LIMA BEANS), AND NUTS	GRAMS OF FIBER
Black beans, ½ cup	8
Bread, 1 slice, white	1
Bread, 1 slice, whole-wheat	2
Bran muffin, 1 medium	3

*Values are for canned or cooked beans.

(Grains, Legumes, and Nuts, *continued*)	GRAMS OF FIBER
Chickpeas, ½ cup	5
Kidney beans, ½ cup	7
Lentils, ½ cup	8
Lima beans, ½ cup	6
Oatmeal, 1 cup cooked	4
Pasta, ½ cup cooked	1
Peanuts, ½ cup	6
Peanut butter, 2 tablespoons, chunky	2
Popcorn, 3 cups air-popped	2
Rice, 1 cup cooked, white	1
Rice, 1 cup cooked, brown	2
Sesame seeds, 2 tablespoons	1
Sunflower seeds, ⅛ cup	2
Tortilla chips, 1 cup (1.5 oz.)	1
Walnuts, ¼ cup chopped	2
Wheat germ, ¼ cup	4

GLYCEMIC INDEX OF SAMPLE FOODS

BEANS

baby lima 32
baked 43
black 30
brown 38
butter 31
chickpeas 33
kidney 27
lentil 30
navy 38
pinto 42
red lentils 27
split peas 32
soy 18

BREADS

bagel 72
croissant 67
kaiser roll 73
pita 57
pumpernickel 49
rye 64
rye, dark 76
rye, whole 50
white 72
whole wheat 72
waffles 76

CEREALS

All-Bran 44
Bran Chex 58
Cheerios 74
corn bran 75
Corn Chex 83
cornflakes 83
Cream of Wheat 66
Crispix 87
Frosted Flakes 55
Grape-Nuts 67
Grape-Nuts Flakes 80
Life 66
muesli 60
NutriGrain 66
oatmeal 49
oatmeal 1 min. 66
puffed wheat 74
puffed rice 90
rice bran 19
Rice Chex 89
Rice Krispies 82
Shredded Wheat 69
Special K 54
Swiss muesli 60
Team 82
Total 76

COOKIES

graham crackers 74
oatmeal 55
shortbread 64
vanilla wafers 77

CRACKERS

Kavli Norwegian 71
rice cakes 82
rye 63
saltine 72
stoned wheat thins 67
water crackers 78

DESSERTS

angel food cake   67

banana bread   47

blueberry muffin   59

bran muffin   60

Danish   59

fruit bread   47

pound cake   54

sponge cake   46

FRUIT

apple   38

apricot, canned   64

apricot, dried   30

apricot jam   55

banana   62

banana, unripe   30

cantaloupe   65

cherries   22

dates, dried   103

fruit cocktail   55

grapefruit   25

grapes   43

kiwi   52

mango   55

orange   43

papaya   58

peach   42

pear   36

pineapple   66

plum   24

raisins   64

strawberries   32

strawberry jam   51

watermelon   72

GRAINS

barley   22

brown rice   59

buckwheat   54

bulgur   47

chickpeas   36

cornmeal   68

couscous   65

hominy   40

millet   75

rice, instant   91

rice, parboiled   47

rye   34

sweet corn   55

wheat, whole   41

white rice   88

white rice, high amylose   59

JUICES

agave nectar   11

apple   41

grapefruit   48

orange   55

pineapple   46

MILK PRODUCTS

chocolate milk   34

ice cream   50

milk   34

pudding   43

soy milk   31

yogurt   38

PASTA

brown rice pasta   92

gnocchi   68

linguine, durum   50

macaroni   46

macaroni & cheese   64

spaghetti   40

spaghetti, protein-enriched   28

USDA FOOD GUIDE PYRAMID

Fats, Oils, & Sweets
Use Sparingly

Milk, Yogurt, & Cheese Group
2–3 Servings

Meat, Poultry, Fish, Dry Beans,
Eggs, & Nuts Group
2–3 Servings

Vegetable Group
3–5 Servings

Fruit Group
2–4 Servings

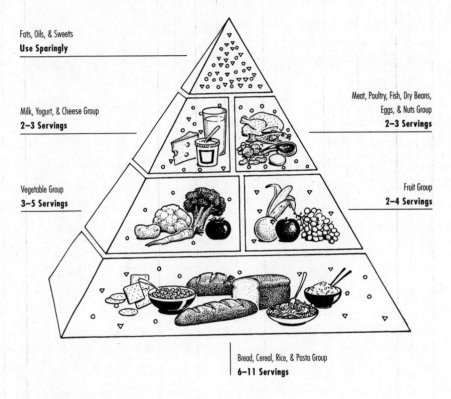

Bread, Cereal, Rice, & Pasta Group
6–11 Servings

Source: USDA

vermicelli 35

vermicelli, rice 58

SWEETS

honey 58

jelly beans 80

Life Savers 70

M&M's chocolate peanut 33

Skittles 70

Snickers 41

Source: The Diabetes Mall, www.diabetes-mall.co

How to Use the Food Guide Pyramid

WHAT COUNTS AS A SERVING?	HOW MANY SERVINGS DO YOU NEED EACH DAY?		
	1,600 CALORIES*	2,200 CALORIES*	2,800 CALORIES*
BREAD, CEREAL, RICE, AND PASTA GROUP	6	9	11

- 1 slice of bread
- About 1 cup of ready-to-eat cereal
- ½ cup of cooked cereal, rice, or pasta

VEGETABLE GROUP	3	4	5

- 1 cup of raw leafy vegetables
- ½ cup of other vegetables—cooked or raw
- ¾ cup of vegetable juice

FRUIT GROUP	2	3	4

- 1 medium apple, banana, orange, pear
- ½ cup of chopped, cooked, or canned fruit
- ¾ cup of fruit juice

MILK, YOGURT, AND CHEESE GROUP— PREFERABLY FAT-FREE OR LOW-FAT	2 or 3†	2 or 3†	2 or 3†

- 1 cup of milk‡ or yogurt
- 1 ½ ounces of natural cheese (such as cheddar)
- 2 ounces of processed cheese (such as American)

MEAT, POULTRY, FISH, DRY BEANS, EGGS, AND NUTS GROUP—PREFERABLY LEAN OR LOW-FAT	2, FOR A TOTAL OF 5 OUNCES	2, FOR A TOTAL OF 6 OUNCES	3, FOR A TOTAL OF 7 OUNCES

- 2–3 ounces of cooked lean meat, poultry, or fish

  These count as 1 ounce of meat:
  - ½ cup of cooked dry beans or tofu
  - 2½-ounce soyburger
  - 1 egg
  - 2 tablespoons of peanut butter
  - ⅓ cup of nuts

*Recommended number of servings depends on your calorie needs:

- 1,600 calories is about right for children ages 2 to 6 years, many sedentary women, and some older adults.
- 2,200 calories is about right for most children over 6, teen girls, active women, and many sedentary men.
- 2,800 calories is about right for teen boys and active men.

†Children and teens ages 9–18 years and adults over age 50 need 3 servings daily; others need 2 servings daily.
‡This includes lactose-free and lactose-reduced milk products. Soy-based beverages with added calcium are an option for those who prefer a non-dairy source of calcium.

NOTE: Many of the serving sizes given above are smaller than those on the Nutrition Facts Label. For example, 1 serving of cooked cereal, rice, or pasta is 1 cup for the label, but only ½ cup for the Pyramid.

Source: USDA

RECOMMENDED DIETARY INTAKES

For more than fifty years, nutrition experts have produced a set of nutrient and energy standards known as the Recommended Dietary Allowances (RDA). A major revision is currently under way to replace the RDA. The revised recommendations are called Dietary Reference Intakes (DRI) and reflect the collaborative efforts of both the United States and Canada. Until 1997, the RDA were the only standards available, and they will continue to serve health professionals until DRI can be established for all nutrients. For this reason, both the 1989 RDA and the 1997 DRI for selected nutrients are presented here.

1989 RECOMMENDED DIETARY ALLOWANCES (RDA)

1997 DIETARY REFERENCE INTAKES (DRI)

AGE (YR)	(kcal) ENERGY	(g) PROTEIN	(µg RE) VITAMIN A	(mg α-TE) VITAMIN E	(µg) VITAMIN K	(mg) VITAMIN C	(mg) THIAMIN	(mg) RIBOFLAVIN	(mg NE) NIACIN	(mg) VITAMIN B_6	(µg) FOLATE	(µg) VITAMIN B_{12}	(mg) IRON	(mg) ZINC	(µg) IODINE	(µg) SELENIUM	(µg) VITAMIN D	(mg) CALCIUM	(mg) PHOSPHORUS	(mg) MAGNESIUM	(mg) FLUORIDE
INFANTS																					
0.0–0.5	650	13	375	3	5	30	0.3	0.4	5	0.3	25	0.3	6	5	40	10	5	210	100	30	0.01
0.5–1.0	850	14	375	4	10	35	0.4	0.5	6	0.6	35	0.5	10	5	50	15	5	270	275	75	0.5
CHILDREN																					
1–3	1,300	16	400	6	15	40	0.7	0.8	9	1.0	50	0.7	10	10	70	20	5	500	460	80	0.7
4–6	1,800	24	500	7	20	45	0.9	1.1	12	1.1	75	1.0	10	10	90	20	5	800	500	130	1.1
7–10	2,000	28	700	7	30	45	1.0	1.2	13	1.4	100	1.4	10	10	120	30					
MALES																					
11–14	2,500	45	1,000	10	45	50	1.3	1.5	17	1.7	150	2.0	12	15	150	40	5	1,300	1,250	240	2.0
15–18	3,000	59	1,000	10	65	60	1.5	1.8	20	2.0	200	2.0	12	15	150	50	5	1,300	1,250	410	3.2
19–24	2,900	58	1,000	10	70	60	1.5	1.7	19	2.0	200	2.0	10	15	150	70	5	1,000	700	400	3.8
25–50	2,900	63	1,000	10	80	60	1.5	1.7	19	2.0	200	2.0	10	15	150	70	5	1,000	700	420	3.8
51+	2,300	63	1,000	10	80	60	1.2	1.4	15	2.0	200	2.0	10	15	150	70	10	1,200	700	420	3.8
																	10	1,200	700	420	3.8

AGE (YR)	(kcal) ENERGY	(g) PROTEIN	(µg RE) VITAMIN A	(mg α-TE) VITAMIN E	(µg) VITAMIN K	(mg) VITAMIN C	(mg) THIAMIN	(mg) RIBOFLAVIN	(mg NE) NIACIN	(mg) VITAMIN B12	(µg) FOLATE	(µg) VITAMIN B12	(mg) IRON	(mg) ZINC	(µg) IODINE	(µg) SELENIUM	(µg) VITAMIN D	(mg) CALCIUM	(mg) PHOSPHORUS	(mg) MAGNESIUM	(mg) FLUORIDE
FEMALES																					
11–14	2,200	46	800	8	45	50	1.1	1.3	15	1.4	150	2.0	15	12	150	45	5	1,300	1,250	240	2.0
15–18	2,200	44	800	8	55	60	1.1	1.3	15	1.5	180	2.0	15	12	150	50	5	1,300	1,250	360	2.9
19–24	2,200	46	800	8	60	60	1.1	1.3	15	1.6	180	2.0	15	12	150	55	5	1,000	700	310	3.1
25–50	2,200	50	800	8	65	60	1.1	1.3	15	1.6	180	2.0	15	12	150	55	5	1,000	700	320	3.1
51+	1,900	50	800	8	65	60	1.0	1.2	13	1.6	180	2.0	10	12	150	55	10	1,200	700	320	3.1
PREGNANT																					
	+300	60	800	10	65	70	1.5	1.6	17	2.2	400	2.2	30	15	175	65	*	*	*	+40	*
LACTATING																					
1st 6 mo.	+500	65	1,300	12	65	95	1.6	1.8	20	2.1	280	2.6	15	19	200	75	*	*	*	*	*
2nd 6 mo.	+500	62	1,200	11	65	90	1.6	1.7	20	2.1	260	2.6	15	16	200	75					

*Values are the same as for other women of comparable age.

Source: RDA reprinted with permission from *Recommended Dietary Allowances,* 10th edition © 1989 by the National Academy of Sciences. Courtesy of the National Academy Press, Washington, D.C.: Committee on Dietary Reference Intakes, *Dietary Reference Intakes for Calcium, Phosphorus, Magnesium, Vitamin D, and Fluoride* (Washington, D.C.: National Academy Press, 1997).

DEFINITIONS USED IN
ADVERTISING AND PACKAGING

The following legal definitions pertain to common terms prevalent in food labeling.

ORGANIC This term has no legal meaning.

NATURAL Refers to a product without additives, artificial flavoring, synthetic ingredients, preservatives, or coloring.

SUGAR-FREE The product is devoid of all simple sugars.

LOW-CALORIE, DIET, REDUCED-CALORIE, OR DIETETIC Contains no more than 40 calories in a single serving or a maximum of 0.4 kcal per gram, or one-third fewer calories than the regular product.

LIGHT OR "LITE" Currently, there are no laws governing the use of these terms.

IMITATION The product is a substitute for and resembles another food but is nutritionally inferior.

SODIUM-FREE Contains less than 5 mg of sodium.

LOW-SODIUM Contains no more than 140 mg of sodium.

VERY-LOW-SODIUM Contains no more than 35 mg of sodium.

REDUCED-SODIUM Sodium is reduced by 75 percent.

FORTIFIED Vitamins and minerals have been added to the product.

ENRICHED Vitamins and iron have been added to the product.

CHOLESTEROL-FREE There is less than 2 mg of cholesterol per serving.

LOW-FAT For meat, fat content does not exceed 10 percent fat by weight; for milk, fat content can range from 0.5 to 2 percent.

FAT-FREE Contains less than 0.5 g of fat per serving.

NEW The product has been changed substantially within the prior six months or is completely new.

NO ARTIFICIAL FLAVORING The product can contain flavors only from naturally occurring products.

NO ARTIFICIAL COLORING The product does not contain one or more of the thirty-three coloring agents that are permitted in food products.

WHEAT Wheat is *one* ingredient of the product.

Source: Katch, Frank I., and William D. McArdle, *Introduction to Nutrition, Exercise and Health*, 4th ed. (Baltimore: Lippincott Williams and Wilkins, 1988).

COMPOSITION OF COMMON FOODS AND BEVERAGES

FOOD	AMOUNT	CALORIES	TOTAL FAT (gm)	SATURATED FAT (gm)	CHOLESTEROL (mg)	SODIUM (mg)	CARBOHYDRATES (gm)		PROTEIN (gm)
							TOTAL	FIBER	
A									
Almonds, dried,									
unblanched	1.0 oz.	168	14.9	1.4	0	3.1	5.8	.8	5.7
Apple, fresh, with									
skin	1 med.	82	.5	.1	0	0	21.2	1.1	.3
Apple juice									
canned or bottled	1 c.	118	.3	.1	0	8	29.3	.5	.2
Applesauce									
sweetened	½ c.	97	.2	trace	0	4	25.5	.6	.2
unsweetened	½ c.	52	.1	trace	0	2	13.8	.6	.2
Apricots									
canned, heavy									
syrup, with skin	1 c.	213	.2	trace	0	10	55.1	1.0	1.4
dried, uncooked	¼ c.	77	.2	trace	0	3	20.1	1.0	1.2
fresh	3	51	.4	trace	0	1	11.8	.6	1.5
Artichokes,									
cooked	½ c.	42	.1	trace	0	79	9.3	1.1	2.9
Asparagus									
canned	1 c.	48	1.8	.3	0	880	6.3	0	5.2
fresh, spears,									
cooked	4 spears	14	.2	trace	0	6	2.5	.5	1.5
frozen cuts and									
tips, cooked	4 spears	17	.2	.1	0	2	2.9	.5	1.8
Avocado									
California	1	305	29.9	4.5	0	21	11.9	3.6	3.6

A dash (–) in a column indicates no reliable data even though component may be present in a measur-able amount.

FOOD	AMOUNT	CALORIES	TOTAL FAT (gm)	SATURATED FAT (gm)	CHOLESTEROL (mg)	SODIUM (mg)	CARBOHYDRATES (gm) TOTAL	CARBOHYDRATES (gm) FIBER	PROTEIN (gm)
B									
Bacon, Canadian,									
broiled or fried,									
drained	2 slices	25	.8	–	10	345	.5	trace	5
Bacon, cured,									
cooked	3 slices	109	9.3	3.3	16	301	.1	0	5.8
Bagel									
egg	1	230	2.5	.5	15	460	41	2.0	9.0
plain	1	210	1.5	0	0	350	40	1.0	10.0
Bamboo shoots,									
raw	1 c.	41	.5	.1	0	6	7.9	1.1	3.9
Bananas, fresh	1 med.	105	.5	.2	0	1	26.6	.6	1.1
Bass, striped,									
plain, cooked	3 oz.	122	3.9	.8	73	75	0	0	20.2
Beans, baked									
in tomato sauce									
with pork	½ c.	123	1.3	.5	9	550	24.3	1.5	6.5
plain or vegetarian	½ c.	116	.6	.1	0	496	25.6	1.4	6.0
Beans, common,									
mature seeds, dry									
KIDNEY, canned,									
solids and liquid	1 c.	203	.8	.1	0	868	37.2	2.5	13.0
PINTO, CALICO, AND									
RED MEXICAN,									
cooked	1 c.	228	.8	.2	0	4	42.8	5.0	13.6
OTHERS, including									
black, brown, and									
bayo, cooked	1 c.	220	.8	.2	0	2	39.6	3.4	14.8
Beans, snap									
(includes Italian,									
yellow, and green)									
cooked	1 c.	44	.4	.1	0	4	9.9	1.8	2.4

FOOD	AMOUNT	CALORIES	TOTAL FAT (gm)	SATURATED FAT (gm)	CHOLESTEROL (mg)	SODIUM (mg)	CARBOHYDRATES (gm)		PROTEIN (gm)
							TOTAL	FIBER	
Beef									
Corned, cooked	3.5 oz.	209	15.8	5.3	82	945	0	0	15.2
Flank steak, choice grade, braised	3 oz.	203	11.5	4.9	59	60	0	0	23.3
Hamburger (ground beef) extra lean, cooked medium	3 oz.	213	13.5	5.3	70	58	0	0	23.8
lean, cooked medium	3 oz.	227	15.4	6.1	73	64	0	0	20.6
regular, cooked medium	3 oz.	241	17.2	6.8	75	69	0	0	20.0
Liver, cooked	3 oz.	134	4.1	1.6	324	58	2.8	0	20.3
Pot roast, choice grade, lean only	3 oz.	195	8.6	3.3	84	55	0	0	27.5
Round entire, choice grade, lean only	3 oz.	162	6.7	2.4	68	53	0	0	23.8
Round eye, choice grade, lean only	3 oz.	153	5.6	2.2	58	52	0	0	24.1
T-bone steak, choice grade, lean only	3 oz.	178	8.7	3.5	67	55	0	0	23.4
Top round (London broil), choice grade, lean only	3 oz.	162	5.4	1.9	70	51	0	0	26.4
Whole ribs, choice grade, lean only	3 oz.	194	11.3	4.8	68	58	0	0	21.7
Beer. *See* Beverages.									
Beets									
boiled, drained	1 c.	73	.3	.1	0	128	16.7	1.3	2.8

FOOD	AMOUNT	CALORIES	TOTAL FAT (gm)	SATURATED FAT (gm)	CHOLESTEROL (mg)	SODIUM (mg)	CARBOHYDRATES (gm) TOTAL	FIBER	PROTEIN (gm)
Beverages—									
See individual fruits for fruit juices.									
Alcoholic									
BEER	12 oz.	146	0	0	0	18	31.2	0	1.1
BEER, LIGHT (low-calorie)	12 oz.	100	0	0	0	11	4.6	0	.7
GIN, RUM, VODKA, WHISKEY	1 oz.	73	0	0	0	.1	0	0	0
WINES, table, all	4 oz.	82	0	0	0	9	1.6	0	.2
Nonalcoholic									
CLUB SODA	12 oz.	0	0	0	0	75	0	0	0
COLAS	12 oz.	152	0	0	0	15	38.5	0	0
CREAM SODAS	12 oz.	189	0	0	0	44	49.3	0	0
GINGER ALE	12 oz.	126	0	0	0	26	32.2	0	0
LEMONADE, frozen, concentrated, diluted	12 oz.	114	.1	.1	0	12	29.1	0	trace
LEMONADE, powder	2 tbsp.	150	0	trace	0	12	39.3	0	4.5
ROOT BEER	12 oz.	152	0	0	0	48	39.3	0	0
SELTZER or sparkling water	12 oz.	0	0	0	0	4	0	0	0
TONIC WATER	12 oz.	125	0	0	0	15	32.6	0	0
Blackberries, boysenberries, dewberries, youngberries, fresh	1 c.	75	.6	0	0	0	18.5	5.9	1.04

FOOD	AMOUNT	CALORIES	TOTAL FAT (gm)	SATURATED FAT (gm)	CHOLESTEROL (mg)	SODIUM (mg)	CARBOHYDRATES (gm)		PROTEIN (gm)
							TOTAL	FIBER	
Black-eyed peas.									
See Cowpeas and									
black-eyed peas.									
Blueberries, fresh	1 c.	81	.6	0	0	9	20.5	1.9	1.0
Bran flakes									
40% bran flakes	1 c.	126	.7	0	0	358	30.1	5.4	4.8
with raisins	1 c.	177	.3	0	0	482	46.1	7.1	4.3
Bread (average loaf)									
FRENCH OR VIENNA	1 slice	70	1	0	0	170	12.0	1.0	2.0
ITALIAN	1 slice	70	1	0	0	170	13.0	1.0	3.0
OATMEAL/OAT-BRAN	1 slice	60	1.0	0	0	160	11.0	1.0	2.0
WHITE ENRICHED	1 slice	70	1.0	0	0	105	12.0	1.0	2.0
WHOLE WHEAT	1 slice	90	1.5	0	0	160	16.0	2.0	4.0
Broccoli									
frozen, chopped,									
cooked	1 c.	56	.2	trace	0	48	10.8	2.4	6.2
whole stalks, fresh,									
cooked	1 stalk	47	.7	.1	0	43	8.5	1.8	5.0
Brussels sprouts,									
fresh, boiled	1 c.	65	.8	.2	0	35	14.5	2.3	4.3
Butter		50	6.0	4.0	20	70	0	0	trace
regular, salted	1 tbsp.	100	11.0	7.0	30	85	0	0	0
Buttermilk,									
cultured, low fat,									
unsalted	1 c.	100	2.3	1.4	10	125	12.0	0	8.3
C									
Cabbage									
cooked, shredded	1 c.	33	.6	.1	0	12	6.7	.9	1.5
raw, shredded	1 c.	18	.2	trace	0	13	3.9	.9	1.0
Cake									
chocolate with									
chocolate icing	1 piece	310	14.0	4.5	20	290	46.0	2.0	3.0
Carrots									
fresh, cooked	1 c.	70	.3	trace	0	103	16.4	2.3	1.7

FOOD	AMOUNT	CALORIES	TOTAL FAT (gm)	SATURATED FAT (gm)	CHOLESTEROL (mg)	SODIUM (mg)	CARBOHYDRATES (gm)		PROTEIN (gm)
							TOTAL	FIBER	
frozen, cooked	1 c.	51	.1	trace	0	84	11.9	1.7	1.7
raw	1 med.	31	.1	trace	0	25	7.1	.7	.7
Cashew nuts									
dry roasted	1 oz.	164	13.3	2.6	0	5	9	.2	4.4
Cauliflower, fresh,									
cooked	1 c.	29	.6	.1	0	19	5.1	1.0	2.3
Celery									
fresh, diced,									
cooked, drained	1 c.	27	.3	.1	0	136	6.0	1.3	1.2
raw	1 stalk	6	trace	trace	0	35	1.5	.3	.3
Cereal: *See* Bran									
flakes; Corn									
products;									
Granola; Oatmeal;									
Oats; Rice									
products; Wheat									
products.									
Chard, Swiss									
fresh, cooked,									
drained	1 c.	35	.2	0	0	314	7.2	1.6	3.3
Cheese									
AMERICAN	1 oz.	104	8.7	5.5	26	397	.4	0	6.2
CHEDDAR									
(domestic)	1 oz.	112	9.2	5.9	29	172	.4	0	6.9
COTTAGE, creamed									
or regular									
(4% milk fat)	½ c.	116	5.1	3.2	17	458	3.0	0	14.1
CREAM		29	0	0	3	144	2	0	4.0
light (neufchatel)	1 oz.	72	6.5	4.1	21	111	.8	0	2.8
regular	1 oz.	97	9.7	6.1	31	82	.7	0	2.1
MOZZARELLA									
with part-skim									
milk	1 oz.	71	4.4	2.8	16	129	.8	0	6.7

FOOD	AMOUNT	CALORIES	TOTAL FAT (gm)	SATURATED FAT (gm)	CHOLESTEROL (mg)	SODIUM (mg)	CARBOHYDRATES (gm) TOTAL	FIBER	PROTEIN (gm)
PARMESAN, grated	1 tbsp.	23	1.5	1.0	4	93	.2	0	2.1
RICOTTA									
with part-skim									
milk	½ c.	171	9.8	6.1	38	155	6.4	0	14.1
with whole milk	½ c.	216	16.1	10.3	63	104	3.8	0	14.0
SWISS	1 oz.	104	7.6	4.9	26	72	.9	0	7.9
Chicken									
skinless, roasted									
breast	½ breast	138	3.0	.8	71	62	0	0	25.8
drumstick	1 drumstick	75	2.5	.7	40	41	0	0	12.3
thigh	1 thigh	110	5.7	1.6	50	46	0	0	13.7
wing	1 wing	43	1.7	.5	18	19	0	0	6.4
with skin, roasted									
breast	½ breast	197	7.7	2.2	84	71	0	0	29.2
drumstick	1 drumstick	114	5.9	1.6	48	47	0	0	14.2
thigh	1 thigh	154	9.7	2.7	58	53	0	0	15.6
wing	1 wing	100	6.7	1.9	29	28	0	0	9.3
Chicken, canned,									
with broth	3 oz.	138	6.7	1.8	–	419	0	0	18.2
Chicken, fried	3 oz.	250	16.0	4.8	50	40	14.0	0	14.0
Chicken liver,									
cooked	¼ c.	54	1.9	.6	218	17.6	.3	0	8.4
Chickpeas, cooked	½ c.	137	2.2	.3	0	6	22.8	2.1	7.4
Chicory									
greens, raw	1 c.	38	.5	.1	0	75	7.8	1.3	2.8
head, bleached									
(Witloof)	½ c.	8	trace	trace	0	1	1.8	0	.4
Chili, canned									
with beans	1 c.	220	7.0	1.5	30	420	15.0	6.0	19.0
Chocolate									
baking, 1 square									
unsweetened	1 oz.	149	15.8	9.3	0	4	8.1	.7	2.9
bittersweet	1 oz.	136	9.8	5.2	0	0	15.6	.7	2.0
semisweet	1 oz.	136	9.1	5.2	.3	0	16.3	.7	2.0
sweet (German)	1 oz.	132	7.7	4.4	0	0	17.6	2.0	2.2

FOOD	AMOUNT	CALORIES	TOTAL FAT (gm)	SATURATED FAT (gm)	CHOLESTEROL (mg)	SODIUM (mg)	CARBOHYDRATES (gm) TOTAL	CARBOHYDRATES (gm) FIBER	PROTEIN (gm)
Chocolate and cocoa flavored beverage powder,									
regular	2–3 tsp.	76	.7	.4	0	46	19.6	.2	.7
Chocolate milk	8 oz.	208	8.5	5.3	30	150	25.8	.2	8.0
Chocolate syrup	1 tbsp.	41	.2	.1	0	18.1	11.1	trace	.4
Clams, cooked	3	123	1.7	.2	56	93	4.3	0	21.3
Cod, cooked	3 oz.	68	.6	.1	36	45	0	0	14.8
Cold cuts.									
See Luncheon meat and cold cuts.									
Coleslaw, cream	½ c.	41	1.5	.2	5	14	7.3	.4	.8
Collards, boiled, drained	1 c.	34	.3	0	0	20	7.6	.6	1.8
Cookies									
CHOCOLATE-CHIP	3	160	8.0	2.5	0	105	21.0	1.0	2.0
GINGERSNAPS	4	120	2.5	.5	0	170	22.0	trace	1.0
GRAHAM CRACKERS, plain	2 whole	120	3.5	.5	0	95	21.0	trace	1.0
OATMEAL	1 large	80	3	.5	0	65	12.0	trace	1.0
OATMEAL RAISIN	2	110	5	1.0	0	70	16.0	1.0	1.0
PEANUT BUTTER	2	130	6.0	1.0	trace	110	19.0	1.0	3.0
Corn, sweet									
canned, cream style	1 c.	180	1.0	.2	0	713	45.0	1.3	4.3
canned, whole kernel, drained	1 c.	135	1.7	.3	0	0	31.0	0	4.3
fresh, kernels or cooked on the cob	1 med. ear or ½ c.	83	1	.2	0	13	19.2	.5	2.5
Corn bread									
home recipe, Southern style	1 piece	161	5.6	–	–	490	22.7	–	5.8

FOOD	AMOUNT	CALORIES	TOTAL FAT (gm)	SATURATED FAT (gm)	CHOLESTEROL (mg)	SODIUM (mg)	CARBOHYDRATES (gm) TOTAL	CARBOHYDRATES (gm) FIBER	PROTEIN (gm)
Corn Chips									
plain	1 oz.	154	9.5	1.3	0	180	16.3	.3	1.9
Crab									
ALASKAN KING,									
cooked	3 oz.	81	1.3	.1	44	893	0	0	16.2
BLUE, crab cakes	3.5 oz.	93	4.5	.9	90	198	.3	trace	12.1
Crackers									
CHEESE	27 small	160	8.0	2.0	0	240	16.0	trace	4.0
GRAHAM.									
See Cookies.									
RYE WAFERS	2	60	0	0	0	75	13.0	4.0	2.0
SALTINES	5	60	1.5	0	0	180	10.0	trace	2.0
THIN WHEAT	16	140	6.0	1	0	120	20.0	2.0	3.0
WATER CRACKER	5	45	0	0	0	90	9.0	1.0	2.0
WHOLE-WHEAT	7	140	5.0	1.0	0	170	21.0	4.0	3.0
Cranberries,									
fresh	1 c.	47	.2	0	0	1	12.1	1.1	.4
Cranberry juice									
cocktail	1 c.	145	.1	0	0	10	37.2	0	.1
Cream									
HALF AND HALF	1 tbsp.	20	1.7	1.1	6	6	.6	0	.4
HEAVY, WHIPPING,									
unwhipped	1 tbsp.	51	5.5	3.4	20	6	.4	0	.3
Cucumber	1 med.								
	(7½"								
	× 2")	40	.3	.1	0	6	8.5	1.8	2.1
D									
Dates	5	115	.2	0	0	1	30.6	.9	.8
Duck									
skinless, cooked	¼ duck	223	12.4	4.7	99	72	0	0	26.1
with skin, cooked	¼ duck	674	56.8	19.4	168	118	0	0	38.0
E									
Eggplant, cooked	1 c.	28	.2	trace	0	3	6.6	1.0	.8

FOOD	AMOUNT	CALORIES	TOTAL FAT (gm)	SATURATED FAT (gm)	CHOLESTEROL (mg)	SODIUM (mg)	CARBOHYDRATES (gm) TOTAL	FIBER	PROTEIN (gm)
Eggs									
fried in butter	1	83	6.4	2.4	246	144	.5	0	5.4
hard- or soft-boiled									
poached, raw	1	79	5.6	1.7	274	69	.6	0	6.1
scrambled	1	93	5.8	2.8	243	151	1.3	0	5.8
white only, raw	1	16	trace	0	0	51	.4	0	3.4
yolk only, raw	1	63	5.6	1.7	272	8	trace	0	2.8
F									
Figs									
canned (light syrup pack), solids and									
liquid	½ c.	86	.1	trace	0	1	22.5	.8	.6
fresh	1 med.	37	.2	trace	0	1	9.6	.6	.4
Fish. *See*									
individual names.									
Frankfurters									
BEEF	1 frank (⅛ lb.)	175	15.8	6.7	34	570	1.0	0	6.7
BEEF, LOW FAT	1 frank (⅛ lb.)	60	1.5	.5	20	480	5.0	0	7.0
CHICKEN/TURKEY	1 frank (⅛ lb.)	142	10.8	3.1	56	660	1.0	0	7.2
French toast, with									
butter	2 slices	377	20.0	8.1	123	543	38.1	.1	11.0
G									
Granola, packaged with almonds and									
seeds	⅓ c.	220	9.0	1.0	0	85	29.0	4.0	6.0
Grapefruit									
fresh—white, pink, or red	½ med.	40	.1	trace	0	0	10.1	.3	.8
Grapefruit juice									
canned, sweetened	1 c.	115	.3	trace	0	5	27.8	0	1.5

FOOD	AMOUNT	CALORIES	TOTAL FAT (gm)	SATURATED FAT (gm)	CHOLESTEROL (mg)	SODIUM (mg)	CARBOHYDRATES (gm) TOTAL	FIBER	PROTEIN (gm)
Grape juice									
canned or bottled	1 c.	153	.2	.1	0	8	37.5	.8	1.5
Grapes									
American type									
(Concord, Delaware,									
Niagara, Catawba,									
scuppernong),									
fresh	1 c.	58	.3	.1	0	2	15.9	.7	.6
H									
Halibut, cooked	3 oz.	116	2.4	.3	34	58	0	0	22.3
Ham. *See* Pork.									
Hamburger.									
See Beef.									
I									
Ice cream and									
frozen custard									
regular									
(approximately									
10% fat)	½ c.	135	7.2	4.5	30	58	15.9	0	2.4
rich									
(approximately									
16% fat)	½ c.	174	11.9	7.4	44	54	16.0	0	2.1
J									
Jams and									
preserves	1 tbsp.	48	trace	trace	0	8	12.9	.1	.1
Jellies	1 tbsp.	51	trace	trace	0	7	13.3	.1	.1
K									
Kale, cooked	1 c.	42	.5	.1	0	30	.6	1.0	2.5
Kiwi	1 med.	47	.3	0	0	4	11.5	.8	.8
Kumquats, fresh	3 small	36	.1	0	0	3	9.4	2.1	.5

FOOD	AMOUNT	CALORIES	TOTAL FAT (gm)	SATURATED FAT (gm)	CHOLESTEROL (mg)	SODIUM (mg)	CARBOHYDRATES (gm) TOTAL	FIBER	PROTEIN (gm)
L									
Lamb									
cubes, for stew, lean									
only, cooked	3 oz.	155	6.1	2.2	75	63	0	0	23.4
ground, cooked	3 oz.	236	16.4	6.8	81	68	0	0	20.7
leg, choice grade, lean									
only, cooked	3 oz.	159	6.4	2.3	74	57	0	0	23.6
loin, choice grade, lean									
only, cooked	3 oz.	168	8.2	3.1	73	55	0	0	22.2
shoulder, choice									
grade, lean only,									
cooked	3 oz.	170	9.0	3.4	73	57	0	0	20.8
Lard	1 tbsp.	116	12.8	5.0	12	trace	0	0	0
Leeks, raw	2	153	.8	.1	0	50	35.3	3.8	3.8
Lemonade.									
See Beverages.									
Lemons, fresh	1 med.	17	.2	trace	0	1	5.5	.2	.6
Lentils, cooked	1 c.	232	.8	.1	0	4	40	5.6	18.4
Lettuce									
BUTTERHEAD									
varieties	1 head	22	.4	.1	0	8	3.8	0	2.2
ICEBERG	1 head	68	1.1	.2	0	47	11.1	2.6	5.2
LOOSE-LEAFED,	2 large								
ROMAINE	leaves	4	.1	trace	0	2	.7	.1	.3
Limes, fresh	1 med.	20	.1	trace	0	1	7.0	.3	.5
Liver. *See* Beef or									
Chicken.									
Lobster, cooked	3 oz.	82	.5	.1	60	317	1.1	0	17.1
Luncheon meat									
and cold cuts									
BOLOGNA, BEEF	1 slice								
	(1 oz.)	89	8.1	3.5	17	280	.2	0	3.5
BOLOGNA, LIGHT	1 slice								
	(1 oz.)	50	4.0	1.5	15	310	1.0	0	3.0

FOOD	AMOUNT	CALORIES	TOTAL FAT (gm)	SATURATED FAT (gm)	CHOLESTEROL (mg)	SODIUM (mg)	CARBOHYDRATES (gm) TOTAL	FIBER	PROTEIN (gm)
CHICKEN ROLL	1 slice (1 oz.)	45	2.1	.6	14	167	.7	0	5.6
HAM, CHOPPED, canned	1 oz.	68	5.4	1.8	14	390	.1	0	4.6
HAM, REGULAR	1 slice (1 oz.)	52	3.0	1.0	16	376	.9	0	5.0
LIVERWURST	1 slice (2/3 oz.)	58	5.1	1.9	28	–	.4	0	4.6
OLIVE LOAF	1 slice (1 oz.)	67	4.7	1.7	11	424	2.6	0	3.4
PASTRAMI	1 slice (1 oz.)	43	2.3	1.0	16.7	320	0	0	5.3
SALAMI, BEEF	1 slice (4/5 oz.)	59	4.7	2.0	14	269	.6	0	3.4
TURKEY OR CHICKEN BREAST	1 slice (4/5 oz.)	23	.3	.1	9	298	0	0	4.7
TURKEY BOLOGNA	1 slice (1 oz.)	57	4.3	–	28	251	.3	0	3.9
TURKEY HAM	1 slice (1 oz.)	37	1.5	.5	–	285	.1	0	5.4
TURKEY PASTRAMI	1 slice (1 oz.)	40	1.8	.5	–	298	.5	0	5.3
TURKEY SALAMI	1 slice (1 oz.)	56	3.9	–	23	287	.2	0	4.7

M

FOOD	AMOUNT	CALORIES	TOTAL FAT (gm)	SATURATED FAT (gm)	CHOLESTEROL (mg)	SODIUM (mg)	CARBOHYDRATES (gm) TOTAL	FIBER	PROTEIN (gm)
Macadamia nuts, dried	1 oz.	200	21.1	3.1	0	1.4	3.9	1.5	2.4
Macaroni. *See* Pasta.									
Mackerel, Atlantic, cooked	3 oz.	218	14.8	3.5	63	69	0	0	19.9
Mangoes, fresh	1 small	135	.6	.1	0	4	35.4	1.7	1.0
Margarine CANOLA, nonfat, soft tub	1 tbsp.	20	2.0	0	0	105	0	0	0

FOOD	AMOUNT	CALORIES	TOTAL FAT (gm)	SATURATED FAT (gm)	CHOLESTEROL (mg)	SODIUM (mg)	CARBOHYDRATES (gm) TOTAL	FIBER	PROTEIN (gm)
CORN, regular, stick or soft tub	1 tbsp.	101	11.3	20	0	140 (av.)	.1	0	.1
SOYBEAN, reduced-fat, stick or soft tub	1 tbsp.	50	6.0	1.0	0	50	0	0	.1
Marmalade	1 tbsp.	49	0	0	0	11	13.3	0	.1
Mayonnaise	1 tbsp.	99	11.0	1.2	–	79	.4	0	.2
Melons, fresh									
CANTALOUPE	½ melon	88	.8	0	0	23	21.0	1.0	2.2
CASABA	1/10 melon	43	.2	0	0	20	10.3	.8	1.5
HONEYDEW	1/10 melon	44	.1	0	0	13	11.5	.8	.6
Milk, cow's,									
Pasteurized or raw									
low fat (1% fat)	1 c.	102	2.6	1.6	10	122	11.7	0	8.0
low fat (2% fat)	1 c.	122	4.6	2.9	20	122	11.7	0	8.1
skim	1 c.	86	.4	.3	5	127	11.9	0	8.4
whole (3.3% fat)	1 c.	484	8.1	5.1	34	120	11.4	0	8.1
See also Buttermilk; Yogurt									
Muffins,									
enriched flour	1	120	0	0	0	220	26.0	trace	2.0
home recipe, blueberry	1	112	3.7	–	–	253	16.8	–	2.9
Mushrooms,									
cultivated commercially, canned, drained	½ c.	19	.2	trace	0	0	3.8	0	1.5
fresh	½ c.	9	.1	trace	0	2	1.6	.3	.7
Mussels, cooked	3 oz.	143	3.8	.8	47	308	6.2	0	19.8
Mustard greens,									
cooked	1 c.	21	.3	trace	0	23	3.0	1.0	3.3
N									
Nectarines, fresh	1 med.	66	.7	0	0	0	15.9	.6	1.2

FOOD	AMOUNT	CALORIES	TOTAL FAT (gm)	SATURATED FAT (gm)	CHOLESTEROL (mg)	SODIUM (mg)	CARBOHYDRATES (gm) TOTAL	FIBER	PROTEIN (gm)
Nuts.									
See individual									
names.									
O									
Oatmeal	1 c.	380	4.0	0	0	0	72.0	6.0	12.0
oatmeal/rolled oats,									
cooked	1 c.	144	2.3	.5	0	2	25.1	.5	6.0
Oils, salad or									
cooking									
CANOLA	1 tbsp.	130	13.5	1.0	0	0	0	0	0
CORN	1 tbsp.	119	13.5	1.7	0	0	0	0	0
OLIVE	1 tbsp.	119	13.5	1.8	0	trace	0	0	0
OTHER VEGETABLES									
(safflower,									
sunflower)	1 tbsp.	119	13.5	1.2	0	0	0	0	0
Okra, cooked	10 pods								
	(3" x ⅜")	36	.2	.1	0	6	8.0	1.0	2.1
Olives									
canned, ripe, small	3	15	1.4	.2	0	114	.8	0	.1
jumbo or									
supercolossal	3	37	3.1	.4	0	408	2.5	0	.5
Orange juice									
canned	1 c.	105	.3	.1	0	5	25.0	.3	1.5
fresh	1 c.	113	.5	.1	0	3	26.0	.3	1.8
Oranges, fresh									
peeled, no seeds,									
all typical									
varietes	1 med.	62	.1	trace	0	0	15.5	.5	1.2
Oysters, cooked	6 oysters	57	2.0	.6	44	176	3.3	0	5.9
P									
Pancakes and									
waffles	2 cakes	170	6.0	1.5	0	490	25.0	trace	3.0
Papayas, fresh	1 fruit	130	.5	.1	0	10	32.7	2.7	2.0

FOOD	AMOUNT	CALORIES	TOTAL FAT (gm)	SATURATED FAT (gm)	CHOLESTEROL (mg)	SODIUM (mg)	CARBOHYDRATES (gm) TOTAL	FIBER	PROTEIN (gm)
Parsley, raw,									
chopped	1 tbsp.	4	.1	0	0	6	.7	.1	.3
Parsnips, cooked	1 c.	135	.5	.1	0	17	32.5	3.7	2.2
Pasta									
cooked	1 c.	201	1.0	.1	0	1	40.4	.1	6.9
egg, cooked	1 c.	222	2.5	.5	55	12	41.3	.2	8.0
spinach, cooked	1 c.	186	.9	.1	0	20	37.4	1.7	6.6
Peaches									
canned in heavy									
syrup	½ c.	93	.1	trace	0	8	25.0	.4	.6
fresh	1 med.	37	.1	trace	0	0	9.7	.5	.6
Peanut butter									
(moderate amounts									
of fat, sweetener,									
and salt)	1 tbsp.	93	7.9	1.5	0	76	3.3	.4	3.9
Peanuts, unroasted,									
unsalted	1 oz.	163	13.8	1.9	0	2	6.0	1.4	6.6
Pears									
canned in heavy									
syrup	½ c.	93	.2	trace	0	6	24.8	.8	.3
fresh, with skin	1 med.	98	.7	trace	0	0	25.2	2.3	.7
Peas									
fresh, cooked,									
drained	1 c.	140	.4	.1	0	5	26.0	3.8	9.0
frozen, cooked,									
drained	1 c.	130	.5	.1	0	145	23.8	3.5	8.6
Pecans, dried	1 oz.	191	19.3	1.5	0	.3	5.2	.5	2.2
Pepperoni.									
See Sausage.									
Peppers									
Hot chili, canned,									
cooked	½ c.	17	.1	trace	0	0	6.1	.8	.6
Perch, cooked	3 oz.	98	1.0	.2	96	66	0	0	20.8
Persimmons	1 small	117	.3	0	0	2	31.0	2.5	1.0

FOOD	AMOUNT	CALORIES	TOTAL FAT (gm)	SATURATED FAT (gm)	CHOLESTEROL (mg)	SODIUM (mg)	CARBOHYDRATES (gm)		PROTEIN (gm)
							TOTAL	FIBER	
Pickles									
Dill	1 large (65 g)	12	.1	trace	0	855	2.7	.4	.4
Sour	1 med. (35 g)	4	.1	trace	0	417	.8	.2	.1
Sweet	1 large (35 g)	40	.1	trace	0	324	11.0	.2	.1
Pies (1 piece equals approx. ⅐ of a 9" pie)									
Apple	1 piece	300	14.0	3.5	0	300	42.0	2.0	2.0
Chocolate cream	1 piece	290	14.0	4.0	0	180	37.0	1.0	2.0
Pecan	1 piece	431	23.6	–	–	228	52.8	–	5.3
Pike, cooked	3 oz.	94	.8	.1	42	41	0	0	20.6
Pineapple									
canned in heavy syrup	2 slices	91	.1	trace	0	1	23.5	.5	.4
fresh, diced	1 c.	75	.6	trace	0	2	19.1	.8	.6
Pineapple juice, canned, unsweetened	1 c.	140	.2	trace	0	3	34.5	.3	.8
Pistachio nuts, dry roasted	1 oz.	173	15.1	1.9	0	2	7.9	.5	4.3
Pita bread									
2-oz. size	1	150	1.0	0	0	290	31.0	1.0	6.0
Pizza, baked	⅛ of a 12" pie								
with cheese	1 slice	139	3.2	1.6	10	333	20.3	.3	7.6
with meat and vegetables	1 slice	185	5.4	1.5	21	384	21.4	.8	13.1
Plums									
canned in heavy syrup	½ c.	111	.1	trace	0	24	28.7	.4	.5
fresh	1 med.	37	.4	trace	0	0	8.9	.4	.5
Pomegrantes, fresh	1 med.	105	.5	0	0	5	26.2	.3	1.5

FOOD	AMOUNT	CALORIES	TOTAL FAT (gm)	SATURATED FAT (gm)	CHOLESTEROL (mg)	SODIUM (mg)	CARBOHYDRATES (gm) TOTAL	FIBER	PROTEIN (gm)
Popcorn									
air-popped	1 c.	31	.3	trace	0	trace	6.2	.3	1.0
microwave, regular	1 c.	33	2.0	.7	0	60	4.0	0	.7
Pork									
BOSTON BLADE, fresh, roasted, lean only	3 oz.	213	14.0	4.8	82	61	0	0	20.3
HAM, CANNED, roasted, extra lean	3 oz.	113	4.1	1.3	25	946	.4	0	17.7
HAM, CURED, fresh, whole, roasted	3 oz.	131	4.6	1.5	46	1106	0	0	20.9
HAM, STEAK, boneless, fresh, extra lean	3 oz.	102	3.6	1.2	38	1058	0	0	16.3
LOIN, fresh, roasted, lean only	3 oz.	200	11.5	4.0	75	58	0	0	22.4
SIRLOIN, fresh, roasted, lean only	3 oz.	196	11.0	3.8	75	52	0	0	22.9
SPARE RIBS, fresh, lean and fat, cooked	3 oz.	331	25.3	9.8	101	78	0	0	24.3
Potato chips									
plain	1 oz.	153	9.9	3.1	0	170	15.1	.5	2.0
Potatoes, white									
baked or microwaved, with skin	1 med.	218	.2	trace	0	16	50.5	1.3	4.6
boiled, with skin	1 med.	119	.1	trace	0	5	27.5	.4	2.6
Pretzels, hard,									
plain	1 oz.	109	1.0	.2	0	490	22.6	.1	2.6
Prune juice	1 c.	178	.1	trace	0	10	43.8	trace	1.5
Prunes									
dried, softened, uncooked	1 c.	398	.8	.1	0	7	105	3.3	4.3

FOOD	AMOUNT	CALORIES	TOTAL FAT (gm)	SATURATED FAT (gm)	CHOLESTEROL (mg)	SODIUM (mg)	CARBOHYDRATES (gm) TOTAL	FIBER	PROTEIN (gm)
R									
Raisins, uncooked	1 c. pressed down	503	.8	.3	0	20	132.5	2.3	5.7
Raspberries									
fresh	1 c.	61	.7	trace	0	0	14.5	3.8	1.1
Rhubarb									
uncooked	1 c.	26	.2	0	0	5	5.5	.9	1.1
Rice									
BROWN, cooked	1 c.	222	1.8	.4	0	10	46.0	.7	5.2
WHITE, enriched, regular, cooked	1 c.	217	.5	.2	0	2	47.0	.2	4.5
See also Wild rice.									
Rolls and buns									
plain	1	119	3.0	–	–	98	19.6	–	2.9
Brown-and-serve-type rolls	1	70	1.0	0	0	350	12.0	1.0	2.0
Frankfurter and hamburger rolls	1	110	2.0	0	0	210	20.0	1.0	4.0
Hard rolls, enriched	1	156	1.6	–	–	313	29.9	–	4.9
S									
Salad Dressings									
BLUE CHEESE	1 tbsp.	78	8.0	1.5	–	–	1.1	trace	.7
FRENCH/RUSSIAN	1 tbsp.	66	6.3	1.5	–	210	2.7	.1	.1
ITALIAN	1 tbsp.	69	7.1	1.0	–	116	1.5	trace	.1
RANCH/CREAMY ITALIAN	1 tbsp.	85	9.0	1.5	2.5	135	1.0	0	0
Salmon, pink									
canned, solids with bone and liquid, no salt added	3 oz.	116	5.1	1.3	–	63	0	0	16.5
fresh, cooked	3 oz.	124	3.7	.6	56	72	0	0	21.3

FOOD	AMOUNT	CALORIES	TOTAL FAT (gm)	SATURATED FAT (gm)	CHOLESTEROL (mg)	SODIUM (mg)	CARBOHYDRATES (gm) TOTAL	FIBER	PROTEIN (gm)
Sauerkraut, canned,									
solids and liquid	1 c.	48	.4	.1	0	1653	10.8	2.8	2.3
Sausage									
BRATWURST, COOKED	1 link	251	21.6	7.8	50	464	1.8	0	11.8
ITALIAN, COOKED	1 link	215	17.1	6.1	52	615	1.0	0	13.3
KNOCKWURST	1 link	205	18.5	6.8	39	673	1.2	0	7.9
PEPPERONI	1 slice	27	2.4	.9	–	113	.2	0	1.2
POLISH-STYLE	½ link	362	31.9	11.4	78	973	1.8	0	15.7
PORK, COOKED	1 link	48	4.1	1.4	11	168	.1	0	2.6
TURKEY	1 link	140	8.0	2.0	70	760	2.0	0	18.0
VIENNA, CANNED	1 link	44	4.0	1.5	8	151	.3	0	1.6
Scallops, raw	5 small	27	.2	trace	10	49	.7	0	5.1
Sea bass, cooked	3 oz.	103	2.2	.5	44	73	0	0	19.7
Sesame seeds,									
dried	1 tbsp.	47	4.4	.6	0	3	.8	.2	2.1
Shrimp, cooked	4 large	90	1.0	.3	177	204	0	0	19.0
Snapper, cooked	3 oz.	106	1.4	.3	39	48	0	0	21.9
Soda. *See* Beverages.									
Sour cream	1 tbsp.	26	2.5	1.6	5	6	.5	0	.4
Soybeans,									
(mature seeds)									
cooked	1 c.	74	4.1	.5	0	9	5.9	1.8	7.7
Spaghetti. *See* Pasta.									
Spinach									
canned, drained	1 c.	49	1.1	.2	0	57	7.2	0	6.0
cooked	1 c.	41	.5	.1	0	125	6.8	1.6	5.4
frozen leaf, boiled,									
drained	1 c.	54	.4	trace	0	165	10.2	2.1	6.0
raw, chopped	1 c.	12	.2	trace	0	44	1.9	.5	1.6
Squash									
SUMMER, all types									
cooked	1 c.	36	.5	.1	0	2	7.7	1.1	1.6
raw	1 c.	26	.3	.1	0	3	5.7	.8	1.6

FOOD	AMOUNT	CALORIES	TOTAL FAT (gm)	SATURATED FAT (gm)	CHOLESTEROL (mg)	SODIUM (mg)	CARBOHYDRATES (gm) TOTAL	FIBER	PROTEIN (gm)
WINTER, all types									
cooked	1 c.	78	1.3	.2	0	2	17.6	1.4	1.8
raw	½ med.								
	squash	43	.2	.1	0	5	10.2	1.6	1.7
ZUCCHINI									
cooked	1 c.	29	.1	trace	0	6	7.0	.9	1.1
frozen, cooked	1 c.	43	.3	.1	0	5	9.0	1.5	3.0
raw	1 c.	18	.1	trace	0	4	3.8	.6	1.6
Steak. *See* Beef.									
Strawberries									
fresh	1 c.	45	.6	trace	0	2	10.4	.7	.9
frozen, sliced,									
sweetened	½ c.	120	.2	trace	0	4	32.4	.8	.6
Sturgeon, cooked	3 oz.	113	4.3	1.0	0	0	0	0	17.3
Sugar									
Beet or cane	1 oz.								
brown	packed	104	0	0	0	11	27.0	0	0
granulated	1 tsp.	15	0	0	0	trace	4.0	0	0
powdered	1 oz.								
	unsifted	58	trace	0	0	trace	14.9	0	0
Sunflower seed									
kernels, dried	1 oz.	163	14.2	1.5	0	1	5.4	1.2	6.5
Sweet potatoes									
baked in skin	1 med.	118	.1	trace	0	0	27.9	.9	2.0
candied	1 piece	144	3.5	1.5	8	74	29.4	.4	.9
Swordfish, cooked	3 oz.	129	4.3	1.2	42	96	0	0	21.2
T									
Tangerines, raw	1 med.	37	.2	trace	0	1	9.3	.3	.5
Tofu									
regular, raw	½ c.	95	6.0	.9	0	8.8	2.4	.1	10.1
Tomato juice,									
canned, regular	8 oz.	21	.1	trace	0	451	5.3	.5	1.0
Tomato paste,									
canned	¼ c.	53	.6	.1	0	40	11.8	.6	2.4

FOOD	AMOUNT	CALORIES	TOTAL FAT (gm)	SATURATED FAT (gm)	CHOLESTEROL (mg)	SODIUM (mg)	CARBOHYDRATES (gm) TOTAL	FIBER	PROTEIN (gm)
Tomato sauce									
canned,									
unseasoned	1 c.	75	.5	.1	trace	1512	18.0	1.8	3.3
Tomatoes (ripe)									
canned, whole	1 c.	50	.5	.1	0	408	10.8	1.3	2.3
cooked	1 c.	68	1.0	.2	0	28	14.5	2.0	2.8
raw	1 med.	26.2	.4	.1	0	11	5.8	.9	1.1
Trout, cooked	3 oz.	158	7.1	1.3	62	56	0	0	22.2
Tuna, canned									
CHUNK LIGHT,									
in oil	3 oz.	165	9.0	1.5	40	375	0	0	20.0
CHUNK LIGHT,									
in water	3 oz.	90	.8	0	40	375	0	0	20.0
Bluefin, fresh,									
cooked	3 oz.	153	5.3	1.3	41	42	0	0	24.9
Turkey									
dark meat, skinless,									
cooked	3 oz.	147	3.9	1.4	102	72	0	0	26.2
dark meat, with									
skin, cooked	3 oz.	165	6.5	1.9	106	69	0	0	25.2
light meat, skinless,									
cooked	3 oz.	127	1.1	.4	78	51	0	0	27.5
light meat, with									
skin, cooked	3 oz.	149	4.1	1.2	86	52	0	0	26.2
V									
Veal									
cubed for stew, lean									
only, cooked	3 oz.	157	3.6	1.1	121	78	0	0	29.2
ground, cooked	3 oz.	143	6.3	2.5	86	69	0	0	20.3
loin, lean only,									
cooked	3 oz.	146	5.8	2.2	88	80	0	0	21.9
sirloin, lean only,									
cooked	3 oz.	140	5.2	2.0	87	71	0	0	21.9
Vegetable									
shortening	1 tbsp.	113	12.8	3.2	–	–	0	0	0

FOOD	AMOUNT	CALORIES	TOTAL FAT (gm)	SATURATED FAT (gm)	CHOLESTEROL (mg)	SODIUM (mg)	CARBOHYDRATES (gm) TOTAL	FIBER	PROTEIN (gm)
W									
Waffles									
frozen	2	200	7.0	1.5	5.0	530	31.0	2.0	4.0
See also Pancakes and waffles.									
Walnuts, English or Persian,									
dried	1 oz.	183	17.7	1.6	0	3	5.2	1.3	4.1
Water chestnuts,									
Chinese, raw	½ c.	66	.1	0	0	9	14.9	.5	.9
Watercress, raw	½ c.	2	trace	trace	0	7	.2	.1	.4
Watermelon	1 c.	51	.6	0	0	3	11.4	.5	1.0
Wheat flour, white,									
all-purpose	1 c.	455	1.3	.3	0	3	95.4	.4	12.9
Wheat germ,									
toasted	⅛ c.	50	1.4	.2	0	1	6.5	.3	3.8
Whitefish, cooked	3 oz.	143	6.3	1.0	64	54	0	0	20.4
Wild rice, cooked	1 c.	168	.5	.1	0	5	35.6	.5	6.7
Wine.									
See Beverages.									
Y									
Yams. *See* Sweet potatoes.									
Yogurt									
fruit or flavored									
low-fat	1 c.	255	2.8	1.8	10	145	47.8	.3	11.0
nonfat, sugar-free	1 c.	100	0	0	5	140	17.0	0	9.0
whole milk	1 c.	138	7.4	4.8	30	104	10.6	0	7.9
Z									
Zucchini. *See* Squash.									

Source: *Random House Webster's Eat Smart Diet and Nutrition Guide,* 2nd ed. (New York: Random House, 1996).

HOW TO READ A FOOD LABEL

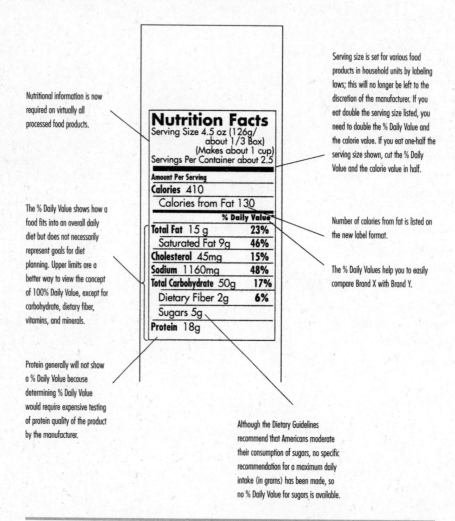

Nutritional information is now required on virtually all processed food products.

Serving size is set for various food products in household units by labeling laws; this will no longer be left to the discretion of the manufacturer. If you eat double the serving size listed, you need to double the % Daily Value and the calorie value. If you eat one-half the serving size shown, cut the % Daily Value and the calorie value in half.

The % Daily Value shows how a food fits into an overall daily diet but does not necessarily represent goals for diet planning. Upper limits are a better way to view the concept of 100% Daily Value, except for carbohydrate, dietary fiber, vitamins, and minerals.

Number of calories from fat is listed on the new label format.

The % Daily Values help you to easily compare Brand X with Brand Y.

Protein generally will not show a % Daily Value because determining % Daily Value would require expensive testing of protein quality of the product by the manufacturer.

Although the Dietary Guidelines recommend that Americans moderate their consumption of sugars, no specific recommendation for a maximum daily intake (in grams) has been made, so no % Daily Value for sugars is available.

Nutrition Facts
Serving Size 4.5 oz (126g/ about 1/3 Box) (Makes about 1 cup)
Servings Per Container about 2.5

Amount Per Serving

Calories 410
   Calories from Fat 130

% Daily Value*

Total Fat 15 g	23%
Saturated Fat 9g	46%
Cholesterol 45mg	15%
Sodium 1160mg	48%
Total Carbohydrate 50g	17%
Dietary Fiber 2g	6%
Sugars 5g	
Protein 18g	

The Nutrition Facts panel on a current food label. The box is broken into two parts: A is the top, and B is the bottom. The % Daily Value listed on the label is the percentage of the generally accepted amount of a nutrient needed daily that is present in 1 serving of the product. You can use the % Daily Values to compare your diet with current nutrition recommendations for certain diet components. Let's consider dietary fiber. Assume that you consume 2,000 kcal. per day, which is the energy intake corresponding to the % Daily Values listed on labels. If the total % Daily Value for dietary fiber in all the foods you eat in one day adds up to 100%, your diet meets the recommendations for dietary fiber.

Many vitamin and mineral amounts no longer need to be listed on the nutrition label. Only Vitamin A, Vitamin C, calcium, and iron remain. The interest in or risk of deficiencies of the other vitamins and minerals is deemed too low to warrant inclusion.

| Vitamin A 10% • Vitamin C 0% |
| Calcium 30% • Iron 15% |

Percent Daily Values are based on a 2,000 calorie diet. Your daily values may be higher or lower depending on your calorie needs:

		Calories: 2,000	2,500
Total Fat	Less than	65g	80g
Sat Fat	Less than	20g	25g
Cholest	Less than	300mg	300mg
Sodium	Less than	2,400mg	2,400mg
Total Carb		300g	375g
Fiber		25g	30g

Some % Daily Value standards, such as grams of total fat, increase as energy intake increases. The % Daily Values on the label are based on a 2,000-kcal. diet. This is important to note if you don't consume at least 2,000 kcal. per day.

Calories per gram:
Fat 9 • Carbohydrate 4
• Protein 4

Labels on larger packages may list the number of calories per gram of fat, carbohydrate, and protein.

INGREDIENTS: WATER, ENRICHED MACARONI (ENRICHED FLOUR [NIACIN, FERROUS SULFATE (IRON), THIAMINE MONONITRATE AND RIBOFLAVIN], EGG WHITE), FLOUR, CHEDDAR CHEESE (MILK, CHEESE CULTURE, SALT, ENZYME), SPICES, MARGARINE (PARTIALLY HYDROGENATED SOYBEAN OIL, WATER, SOY LECITHIN, MONO- AND DIGLYCERIDES, BETA CARO- TENE FOR COLOR, VITAMIN A PALMITATE), AND MALTODEXTRIN.

Ingredients, listed in descending order by weight, will appear here or in another place on the package. The sources of some ingredients, such as certain flavorings, will be stated by name to help people better identify ingredients that they avoid for health, religious, or other reasons.

Source: Wardlaw, Gordon M., *Contemporary Nutrition*, 4th ed. (New York: McGraw Hill Companies, Inc., 2000).

CALORIC EXPENDITURE DURING VARIOUS ACTIVITIES

ACTIVITY	CAL/MIN*
Sleeping	1.2
Resting in bed	1.3
Sitting, normally	1.3
Sitting, reading	1.3
Lying, quietly	1.3
Sitting, eating	1.5
Sitting, playing cards	1.5
Standing, normally	1.5
Classwork, lecture (listening)	1.7
Conversing	1.8
Personal toilet	2.0
Sitting, writing	2.6
Standing, light activity	2.6
Washing and dressing	2.6
Washing and shaving	2.6
Driving a car	2.8
Washing clothes	3.1
Walking indoors	3.1
Shining shoes	3.2
Making bed	3.4
Dressing	3.4
Showering	3.4
Driving motorcycle	3.4

*Depends on efficiency and body size. Add 10 percent for each 15 lb. over 150; subtract 10 percent for each 15 lb. under 150.

ACTIVITY	CAL/MIN
Metalworking	3.5
House painting	3.5
Cleaning windows	3.7
Carpentry	3.8
Farming chores	3.8
Sweeping floors	3.9
Plastering walls	4.1
Repairing trucks and automobiles	4.2
Ironing clothes	4.2
Farming, planting, hoeing, raking	4.7
Mixing cement	4.7
Mopping floors	4.9
Repaving roads	5.0
Gardening, weeding	5.6
Stacking lumber	5.8
Sawing with chain saw	6.2
Working with stone, masonry	6.3
Working with pick and shovel	6.7
Farming, haying, plowing with horse	6.7
Shoveling (miners)	6.8
Shoveling snow	7.5
Walking down stairs	7.1
Chopping wood	7.5
Sawing with crosscut saw	7.5–10.5
Tree felling (ax)	8.4–12.7
Gardening, digging	8.6
Walking up stairs	10.0–18.0
Playing pool or billiards	1.8
Canoeing, 2.5 mph–4.0 mph	3.0–7.0

ACTIVITY	CAL/MIN
Playing volleyball, recreational to competitive	3.5–8.0
Golfing, foursome to twosome	3.7–5.0
Pitching horseshoes	3.8
Playing baseball (except pitcher)	4.7
Playing Ping-Pong or table tennis	4.9–7.0
Practicing calisthenics	5.0
Rowing, pleasure to vigorous	5.0–15.0
Cycling, easy to hard	5.0–15.0
Skating, recreational to vigorous	5.0–15.0
Practicing archery	5.2
Playing badminton, recreational to competitive	5.2–10.0
Playing basketball, half or full court (more for fast break)	6.0–9.0
Bowling (while active)	7.0
Playing tennis, recreational to competitive	7.0–11.0
Waterskiing	8.0
Playing soccer	9.0
Snowshoeing (2.5 mph)	9.0
Slide board	9.0–13.0
Playing handball or squash	10.0
Mountain climbing	10.0–15.0
Skipping rope	10.0–15.0
Practicing judo or karate	13.0
Playing football (while active)	13.3
Wrestling	14.4
Skiing	
Moderate to steep	8.0–20.0

ACTIVITY	CAL/MIN
Downhill racing	16.5
Cross-country; 3–10 mph	9.0–20.0
Swimming	
Leisurely	6.0
Crawl, 25–50 yd/min.	6.0–12.5
Butterfly, 50 yd/min.	14.0
Backstroke, 25–50 yd/min.	6.0–12.5
Breaststroke, 25–50 yd/min.	6.0–12.5
Sidestroke, 40 yd/min.	11.0
Dancing	
Modern, moderate to vigorous	4.2–5.7
Ballroom, waltz to rumba	5.7–7.0
Square	7.7
Walking	
Road or field (3.5 mph)	5.6–7.0
Snow, hard to soft (2.5–3.5 mph)	10.0–20.0
Uphill, 15 percent grade (3.5 mph)	8.0–15.0
Downhill, 5–10 percent grade (2.5 mph)	3.5–3.7
15–20 percent grade (2.5 mph)	3.7–4.3
Hiking, 40-lb. pack (3.0 mph)	6.8
Running	
12-min. mile (5 mph)	10.0
8-min. mile (7.5 mph)	15.0
6-min. mile (10 mph)	20.0
5-min. mile (12 mph)	25.0

Source: Sharkey, Brian J., PhD., *Fitness and Health,* 4th ed. (Champaign: Human Kinetics, 1997).

OTHER SOURCES OF INFORMATION AND SUPPORT

American Dietetic Association
www.eatright.org
American Dietetic Association
216 W. Jackson Boulevard
Chicago, Illinois 60606-6995
1-312-899-0040

United States Department of Agriculture
www.usda.gov
USDA Food and Nutrition Service
3101 Park Center Drive
Alexandria, Virginia 22302
Administrator's Office, Room 906
1-703-305-2060

National Institutes of Health
www.nih.gov
National Institutes of Health (NIH)
Bethesda, Maryland 20892
1-877-946-4627

American Obesity Association
www.obesity.org
American Obesity Association
1250 24th Street NW
Suite 300
Washington, D.C. 20037
1-800-98-OBESE (1-800-986-2373)
or 202-776-7711

American Heart Association
www.americanheart.org
National Center Mailing Address
American Heart Association
National Center
7272 Greenville Avenue
Dallas, Texas 75231
1-800-242-8721

American Diabetes Association
www.diabetes.org
American Diabetes Association
ATTN: Customer Service
1701 North Beauregard Street
Alexandria, Virginia 22311
1-800-DIABETES (1-800-342-2383)

BIBLIOGRAPHY

Books

Atkins, Robert C., M.D., *Dr. Atkin's Diet Revolution* (New York: Bantam, 1972).

Brody, Tom, *Nutritional Biochemistry,* 2nd ed (Academic Press, 1999).

Cooper, Kenneth H., M.D., M.PH., *The Aerobics Program for Total Well-Being* (New York: Bantam Books, 1982).

Hensrud, Donald D., M.D., *Mayo Clinic on Healthy Weight* (New York: Kensington Publishing Corporation, 2000).

Katch, Frank I., and McArdle, William D., *Introduction to Nutrition, Exercise, and Health,* 4th ed. (Baltimore: Lippincott Williams and Wilkins, 1988).

Mathews, Christopher K., and van Holde, K. E., *Biochemistry* (Redwood City, Calif.: Benjamin/Cummings Publishing Company, 1990).

McArdle, William D., Katch, Frank I., and Katch, Victor L., *Exercise Physiology: Energy, Nutrition, and Human Performance,* 4th ed. (New York: Lippincott Williams and Wilkins, 1996).

Paulsen, Barbara, *The Diet Advisor* (New York: Time-Life Books, 2000).

Rolls, Barbara, Ph.D., and Barnett, Robert, *Volumetrics Weight-Control Plan* (New York: HarperCollins, 2000).

Sears, Barry, Ph.D., *The Zone* (New York: HarperCollins, 1995).

Sharkey, Brian J., PhD., *Fitness and Health,* 4th ed. (Champaign: Human Kinetics, 1997).

Sizer, Frances, and Whitney, Eleanor, *Nutrition: Concepts and Controversies,* 8th ed. (Stamford: Wadsworth/Thomson Learning, 2000).

Steward, H. Leighton, Bethea, Morrison C., Nadrews, Sam S., Brennan, Ralph O., and Balart, Luis A. , *Sugar Busters!: Cut Sugar to Trim Fat* (New York: Ballantine, 1998).

Tarnower, Herman, and Baker, Samm Sinclair *Complete Scarsdale Medical Diet*

Plus Dr. Tarnower's Lifetime Keep-Slim Program (New York: Bantam Books, 1995).

Wardlaw, Gordon M., *Contemporary Nutrition: Issues and Insights*, 4th ed. (New York: The McGraw-Hill Companies, Inc., 2000).

Studies/Articles

The American Dietetics' Association Food and Nutrition Guide.

Willett, W.C., Dietz, W. H., and Colditz, G. A., "Guidelines for Healthy Weight," *New England Journal of Medicine* 341 (1999): 427–34.

National Institutes of Health, "Clinical Guidelines on the Identification, Evaluation, and Treatment of Overweight and Obesity in Adults" (September 1998).

U.S. Department of Health and Human Services, "Physical Activity and Health: A Report of the Surgeon General" (Atlanta, GA.: Centers for Disease Control and Prevention, National Center for Chronic Disease Prevention and Health Promotion, 1996).

Paffenbarger, R. S., Hyde, R. T., Wing, A. L., et al., "The Association of Changes in Physical-Activity Level and Other Lifestyle Characteristics with Mortality Among Men," *New England Journal of Medicine* 328, no. 8 (1993): 538–45.

Sherman, S. E., D'Agostino, R. B., Cobb, J. L., et al., "Physical Activity and Mortality in Women in the Framingham Heart Study," *American Heart Journal* 128, no. 5 (1994): 879–84.

Pate, R. R., Pratt, M., Blair, S. N., et al. "Physical Activity and Public Health: A Recommendation from the Centers for Disease Control and Prevention and the American College of Sports Medicine," *Journal of the American Medical Association* 273, no. 5 (1995): 402–407.

USDA and U.S. Department of Health and Human Services, *Dietary Guidelines for Americans*, 5th ed. (USDA Home and Garden Bulletin No. 232. Washington, D.C.: USDA, 2000).

USDA, *The Food Guide Pyramid* (USDA Home and Garden Bulletin No. 252. Washington, D.C.: USDA, 1992).

Flegal, K. M., Carroll, M.D., Kuczmarski, R. J., et al, "Overweight and Obesity in the United States: Prevalence and Trends, 1960–1994," *International Journal of Obesity* 22, no. 1 (1998): 39–47.

NIH, "Clinical Guideline on the Identification, Evaluation and Treatment of Overweight and Obesity in Adults—The Evidence Report," *Obesity Research* 6 (suppl. 2, 1998): 51S–209S.

PHS, *The Surgeon General's Report on Nutrition and Health* (DHHS Pub. No. [PHS] 88050210, Washington, D.C.: HHS, 1988).

INDEX

ABOUT THE AUTHOR

IAN K. SMITH, M.D., is a medical/health reporter for NBC's *Nightly News* and the *Today* show. He also writes a weekly health column for the New York *Daily News* and is a medical columnist for *Time* magazine. Dr. Smith graduated from Harvard University and earned a master's degree in science education from Columbia University. He attended Dartmouth Medical School and the University of Chicago Pritzker School of Medicine. He is also the author of *Dr. Ian Smith's Guide to Medical Websites*. Dr. Smith currently resides in Manhattan.

ABOUT THE TYPE

This book was set in ITC New Baskerville, a typeface based on the design by John Baskerville. The original was cut by John Handy in 1750. Noted for its high contrast and sparkly look, it saw a renewed popularity when the Lanston Monotype Corporation of London revived the classic Roman face in 1923. The Mergenthaler Linotype Company in England and the United States cut a version of Baskerville in 1931, making it one of the most widely used typefaces today.